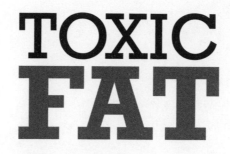

TOXIC FAT

TOXIC FAT

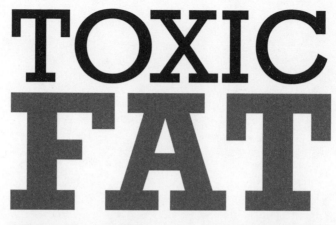

WHEN GOOD FAT TURNS BAD

Barry Sears, Ph.D.

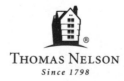

THOMAS NELSON
Since 1798

NASHVILLE   DALLAS   MEXICO CITY   RIO DE JANEIRO   BEIJING

Published in Nashville, Tennessee, by Thomas Nelson. Thomas Nelson is a registered trademark of Thomas Nelson, Inc.

Thomas Nelson, Inc. titles may be purchased in bulk for educational, business, fund-raising, or sales promotional use. For information, please e-mail SpecialMarkets@ThomasNelson.com.

Library of Congress Cataloging-in-Publication Data

Sears, Barry, 1947–
  Toxic fat : when good fat turns bad / Barry Sears.
      p. cm.
  Includes bibliographical references.
  ISBN 978-1-4016-0429-5 (hardcover)
  1. Obesity. 2. Inflammation. 3. Metabolic syndrome. 4. Lipids—Metabolism—Disorders. I. Title.
  RC628.S412 2008
  616.3'98—dc22   2008027184

Printed in the United States of America

08 09 10 11 12 13 QW 6 5 4 3 2 1

Contents

Contents

Introduction

SOMETHING IS TERRIBLY WRONG WITH AMERICA. YOU ONLY HAVE TO walk down the streets to see the surging epidemic of obesity. However, this epidemic is far more complex than simply the result of sloth and gluttony. After years of studying the problem, I have concluded that we can view obesity as a form of "cancer" driven by inflammation.

Obesity can be viewed as an inflammation-induced cancer that can be either benign or malignant. You can live with a benign fat tumor for a long time, but a malignant tumor will kill you. The reason is that a malignant fat tumor is one that rapidly spreads the molecular building block (toxic fat) of inflammation from your fat cells to every organ in your body. When this occurs, you have what I have termed *Toxic Fat Syndrome*.

The first sign that you have a benign fat tumor in your body is the accumulation of excess body fat. However, it is only when this tumor starts to spread toxic fat into the bloodstream that the linkage between obesity and chronic disease begins to occur. The first clinical sign for many people is the development of a cluster of metabolic disturbances (high triglycerides, low HDL cholesterol, and high insulin levels) known as metabolic syndrome. None of these is classified as a disease, but if metabolic syndrome is left untreated, it often develops into type 2 diabetes within about eight to ten years.

But this is only the beginning of the unraveling of your health. This spreading toxic fat that was initially safely contained in your fat cells can now attack every organ system in your body, ranging from the heart to the immune system and the brain. And when enough damage is done, we call it heart disease, cancer, or Alzheimer's.

The causes of this increasingly inflammatory assault of toxic fat on the organs are changes in our diet within the last few decades. No one specific dietary change has caused this increased formation of toxic fat. It's due to a confluence of several dietary factors that have come together at the same time, which I call the Perfect Nutritional Storm. It first appeared in America twenty-five years ago and is now spreading across the world.

This Perfect Nutritional Storm has brought a flood of increased toxic fat, and our epidemic of obesity is a direct result. Initially, increased weight acts as a protective mechanism to prevent the spread of the increased toxic fat into the bloodstream. But under the right circumstances, this encapsulated toxic fat begins to escape and becomes the foundation for the corresponding epidemic of Toxic Fat Syndrome that results in the acceleration of the development of chronic disease. America now ranks twenty-second in the world in wellness, despite our massive amounts of health-care spending. Our epidemic of Toxic Fat Syndrome is the cause.

We know obesity when we see it, but how do we measure toxic fat and the inflammation that comes with it? One parameter might be pain associated with chronic disease. However, chronic disease takes years, if not decades, to develop, and only then does pain begin to emerge. What if there is another type of inflammation that has no associated pain yet is caused by increasing levels of toxic fat in the blood? This would be silent inflammation that drives Toxic Fat Syndrome. It is the increasing levels of silent inflammation that cause us to move from wellness toward chronic disease. You don't yet have enough accumulated organ damage to be considered ill or have a diagnosis of a chronic disease from your doctor, but you are definitely not well.

This book is extremely controversial for three reasons:

1. Being overweight or obese is not your fault. Nor is it a consequence of being morally inferior. It is due to the adverse interaction of your genes with radical changes that have taken place in the American diet over the past twenty-five years.
2. If you have a chronic disease (diabetes, heart disease, arthritis, cancer, or a neurological disorder), it's quite likely that a major underlying cause of your current condition comes from seemingly well-meaning governmental agricultural programs initiated more than thirty years ago.
3. Everything you have heard about the "cause" and the "cure" for the current obesity epidemic is probably dead wrong.

These are pretty powerful statements. That's why this book has a lot of science to support my positions. Although much of this information is known only to a handful of medical researchers, I have tried to make it digestible for the nonscientist. I guarantee it is well worth your effort to stay with me as I explain the real facts behind our obesity epidemic; because by the end of the book, you will come to understand that your personal battle against toxic fat may be the most important factor that determines the quality of the rest of your life.

Toxic Fat Syndrome is caused by your diet, and fighting it is a lifelong struggle. The more we begin to understand the genetics of the human body, the more we understand how certain dietary components can activate the most primitive parts of our immune system to cause an increase in silent inflammation. In the past twenty-five years, the American diet has become more pro-inflammatory, and has fueled our current epidemics of obesity and diabetes. This increased inflammation represents the ultimate cause for the growing loss of wellness in this country. Even more frightening is the fact that we are now exporting this Toxic Fat Syndrome epidemic around the world.

This book describes what caused this epidemic of Toxic Fat Syndrome, why it is spreading, and what the consequences will be if it is left unchecked. It presents a clinically proven approach that combines the anti-inflammatory Zone Diet—a simple balance of low-fat protein and low glycemic-load carbohydrates—plus high-dose fish oil to reverse this inflammation epidemic that has resulted in the spread of obesity and the acceleration of chronic disease.

I hope that you will use this book as a clear dietary road map back to wellness—one that doesn't sentence you to a lifetime of expensive drugs or medical care to save you from yourself. It depends upon your desire to regain control of your future health using the food that you eat. Your personal future depends on your ability to reduce toxic fat and thus reverse Toxic Fat Syndrome.

It's easy, and you can see results in less than thirty days.

CHAPTER 1

The Real Epidemic Behind the Obesity Crisis

IRE WARNINGS APPEAR EVERY DAY. GOVERNMENT OFFICIALS make impressive speeches about its dangers. Task forces are being assembled. Massive funds are promised. What is the cause of this grave concern? Are we going to war again? Yes, we are, and the enemy is obesity.

Many of us have battled extra pounds, and it hasn't been a particularly successful battle. People without weight problems seem to think the cause of obesity is simply sloth and gluttony. I believe the root cause is something far more insidious, which I liken to a cancer that threatens every organ in the body. And in many people, accumulation of excess body fat initially represents a biological defense response trying to protect our bodies from this potential "cancer."

This means that all of our efforts to follow the advice of simple slogans such as "eat less and exercise more" may be meaningless, and our current obesity crisis will continue unabated, if not accelerate—unless we attack the problem from a different perspective.

What we see as our current obesity epidemic is only the tip of a vastly more dangerous epidemic of inflammation—not the type of inflammation we can feel, but inflammation that lies below the perception of pain. I call this silent inflammation. It is this type of inflammation that is driving our obesity epidemic and a wide number of other chronic diseases. The underlying cause of chronic disease comes from the increased production of a natural fatty acid called arachidonic acid (AA), which can be incredibly toxic at high enough concentrations. This is the toxic fat that is key to not only understanding our obesity epidemic but also providing the linkage between obesity and chronic disease. Oddly enough, accumulation of excess body fat is initially your body's attempt to protect you, by encapsulating or trapping this toxic fat in your fat cells so it doesn't attack your other organs. The problem is that the toxic fat doesn't stay trapped in your fat cells forever. Once it begins to spill over into the blood, you have Toxic Fat Syndrome. The resulting health problems associated with Toxic Fat Syndrome are relentless.

Toxic Fat Syndrome is the real epidemic that threatens our health. After years of inflammatory assaults caused by toxic fat, enough damage occurs to a particular organ that we call it chronic disease. That chronic disease might be heart disease, diabetes, cancer, or even Alzheimer's, but it had its start as Toxic Fat Syndrome.

Toxic Fat Syndrome has similarities to Toxic Shock Syndrome, which showed up in 1980, apparently caused by super-absorbent tampons. Both syndromes cause the body's normal immune system to go into overdrive attacking itself. But Toxic Fat Syndrome causes organ damage at a much slower rate. The vast majority of Americans suffer from Toxic Fat Syndrome and don't know it—and it is all caused by what you eat.

If the flow of toxic fat into the bloodstream is left unchecked, the result is a checklist of the chronic diseases that represent the bulk of our current health-care expenditures, such as:

- Allergies
- Asthma
- Autoimmune diseases (arthritis, lupus, and others)
- Cancer
- Heart disease
- Inflammatory diseases (Crohn's disease, ulcerative colitis, and others)
- Neurological disorders (Alzheimer's, depression, ADHD, and others)
- Type 2 diabetes

The appearance of each of these chronic diseases can be viewed as different manifestations of Toxic Fat Syndrome. Your genetics determine which organ in your body is affected first. But if you have one chronic condition associated with Toxic Fat Syndrome, the others are probably not too far behind.

You can't tell if people have Toxic Fat Syndrome just by looking at them. Only the blood will reveal it because the appearance of toxic fat in the bloodstream is the first sign you are no longer well and are headed more rapidly toward any one of many chronic conditions associated with Toxic Fat Syndrome. But don't despair; you can begin to reverse Toxic Fat Syndrome in less than thirty days if you follow the easy dietary prescriptions I describe in this book.

Even though an increase in obesity may initially be your body's way to try to prevent the spread of toxic fat to other organs, these storage sites for toxic fat can also be staging areas for its future malignant spread throughout the body. The sooner you realize that you have circulating toxic fat, the more easily it can be reversed before there is too much organ damage. The solution to Toxic Fat Syndrome is the same factor that caused it in the first place—your diet. What is required is an anti-inflammatory diet to combat the effects of a growing Perfect Nutritional Storm. The dietary solution to the Perfect Nutritional Storm is simple, and it can be followed for a lifetime. The end result will be a longer and better life.

CHAPTER 2

The Perfect Nutritional Storm

TOXIC FAT SYNDROME IN AMERICA DIDN'T APPEAR OVERNIGHT— and no one single dietary factor was the cause. This health crisis was generated only when three distinct dietary factors came together simultaneously, creating the Perfect Nutritional Storm. The three food factors needed for this Perfect Nutritional Storm are:

➤ Cheap refined carbohydrates
➤ Cheap vegetable oil
➤ Decreased consumption of fish oil

This occurred first in America in the 1980s and now is spreading worldwide through growing use of cheap bulk-food commodities that are the foundation of all processed foods. Nowhere in the world is the know-how of making and marketing cheap, palatable processed foods more concentrated than in America, and that's why Toxic Fat Syndrome first appeared here.

When all three of these factors occur together, you have the ingredients for an epidemic of inflammation driven by increasing levels of toxic fat in the blood. It's this increased inflammation that has caused our current twin epidemics of obesity and type 2 diabetes. But these two diseases are only the most obvious initial consequences of Toxic Fat Syndrome. Other conditions associated with Toxic Fat Syndrome are heart disease, cancer, neurological disorders, autoimmune disorders, asthma, allergies, and many more. These conditions are appearing at earlier ages in Americans, in spite of the massive level of fiscal resources we spend on health care.

So let's examine these three components of the Perfect Nutritional Storm, because each appears innocuous until they all come together.

Cheap Carbohydrates

Why are cheap carbohydrates, such as grains, a problem? After all, isn't bread considered the "staff of life"? The rapid rise of industrialized farming in the 1970s made grains one of the most inexpensive sources of calories known. Unfortunately, eating too many of these cheap carbohydrates can actually shorten our lifespan. The reason is that consumption of excess amounts of these high glycemic-load carbohydrates (especially refined carbohydrates) causes the body to produce excess insulin. As I explained in one of my earlier books, *The Anti-Aging Zone*, excess levels of insulin speed up the aging process as well as increase the potential production of more toxic fat.

An excess supply of food (even carbohydrates) has been a relatively new phenomenon in human history. In the past, it took a lot of effort to grow food; even more effort was needed to cook and prepare it, and food was perishable. All of this began to change in the twentieth century with the introduction of processed foods.

The first of these industrially processed foods was breakfast cereal. Just add milk, and instantaneously you have a meal. (Of course, you had to have access to milk.) Next were the highly portable sources of calories, such as sugar-laden soft drinks and candy bars, that again relied on relatively cheap carbohydrates, both with a long shelf life (pretty important if you didn't have a refrigerator). But the trend really picked up after World War II, when food processing began to take off as people had less time to prepare meals at home.

The American food-processing industry remains the world leader in making an amazing variety of highly palatable junk foods composed primarily of cheap carbohydrates. The emergence of fast-food restaurants meant you no longer needed to eat your meals at home. These meals included lots of cheap carbohydrates. Even food items such as breakfast cereals, bread, and pasta are nothing more than simple forms of processed foods made possible by the advent of cheap refined carbohydrates.

But this agricultural transformation that increased the levels of insulin that resulted from increased carbohydrate consumption was not sufficient in itself to cause a rapid rise in the formation of toxic fat. For that you needed the other shoe to drop, and that was accomplished through another recent food phenomenon—cheap seed oils, rich in omega-6 fatty acids.

Cheap Vegetable Oils

In the past, vegetable seed oils were very expensive to produce. Throughout history most fats came from lard, butter, or olive oil. None of these traditional fats had much impact on inflammation because they contain very limited amounts of omega-6 fatty acids. However, by the 1920s the industrial processing of vegetable seeds, such as soybeans and corn (basically using gasoline as an extracting solvent), began to make vegetable oil production much less expensive. And those vegetable oils (primarily corn and soybean) are rich in certain types of polyunsaturated fatty acids known as omega-6 fatty acids—which are the building blocks for the potential production of increased amounts of toxic fat. However, it is only when you begin to mix excess insulin (coming from cheap carbohydrates) with excess omega-6 fatty acids (coming from cheap vegetable oils) that you get increased production of toxic fat.

If this story has a pivotal character, it is Earl Butz, who headed the Department of Agriculture during the Nixon administration. He did more to unleash the tsunami of cheap carbohydrates and cheap vegetable oils than any other person in history. Before Butz, if American farmers produced too much food, they were paid subsidies to remove parts of their acreage from production until the prices went back up. This was a tactic left over from the Depression when overfarming was destroying croplands. Butz took the opposite approach—he wanted American farmers to put the pedal to the metal to maximize food production for export sales to help support a weakening dollar caused by the first oil shock in the early 1970s. New genetic strains of food that had a higher carbohydrate content were now available. Unfortunately, they required high levels of fertilizers and herbicides to maintain the increased output. This was the birth of agribusiness as the farmers became dependent on the chemical companies to increase their productivity to service new export markets. Now grain production could be pushed to the maximum. If farmers produced too much, the government would now pay them a subsidy based on a set market price, no matter how low the real crop price dropped.

It turned out that only crops that could produce the most calories per acre of land would benefit from this program. That left out fruits and vegetables, but it was ideally suited for two crops that could be produced with ruthless abandon by applying industrial farming techniques: corn and soybeans.

Not only were these crops extremely efficient for industrial-sized farms, but with the growing sophistication of the food-processing industry, these crops provided a wide variety of different components that could be used to make hundreds of new, more valuable ingredients. From corn came corn syrup (and its biotechnology cousin, high-fructose corn syrup), corn oil, industrial chemicals, and alcohol as a gasoline replacement. Soybeans were even more abundant, producing not only soybean oil and protein but also even more useful industrial chemicals.

By combining increasingly cheap corn and soybeans as feedlot ingredients, you can produce less-expensive beef, pork, and chicken. These traditional farm animals were now becoming industrial manufacturing factories to convert cheap corn and soybeans (all supported by governmental subsidies) into inexpensive meat products for the fast-food and restaurant business. In 2007, the subsidies for corn and soybeans were nearly $20 billion per year while government support for fruits and vegetables was virtually zero.

One of the first recipients of this government largesse was the processed food industry, which could now convert ever-increasingly inexpensive raw materials into highly portable, convenient, palatable, and incredibly cheap foods. In a very short period of time, traditional American agriculture became an industrial complex that was the foremost low-cost producer in the world. Just as manufacturing is moving to China because of its low labor costs, America has become the low-cost producer of the key raw materials necessary to make processed foods for the world. And nowhere in the world is the technological expertise more sophisticated to make processed foods than in the United States.

While neither cheap carbohydrates nor cheap vegetable oils alone were sufficient to make the current epidemic of inflammation possible, combining them in processed foods was like adding a lighted match to a vat of gasoline. All grains and starches are composed of pure glucose held together by very weak chemical bonds that are rapidly broken during digestion. The released glucose rapidly enters the bloodstream to cause the release of the hormone insulin. Increasing levels of insulin drive omega-6 fatty acids from vegetable oils to make more arachidonic acid (toxic fat)—the building block for incredibly powerful inflammatory hormones known as eicosanoids. In other words, bad things begin to happen.

But one more change in our food supply had to occur before the full impact of the epidemic of silent inflammation could emerge.

Decrease in Fish Oil Consumption

Mankind has always had a trump card against diet-induced inflammation: high consumption of long-chain polyunsaturated omega-3 fatty acids from fish and fish oils. Although very close in structure to omega-6 fatty acids, these omega-3 fatty acids in high enough concentrations are powerful anti-inflammatory agents. So even with the growing consumption of cheap carbohydrates and cheap vegetable oils, adequate intake of these omega-3 fatty acids could keep diet-induced inflammation in check. Unfortunately in America, just as the intake of cheap carbohydrates and cheap vegetable oils was increasing, the consumption of long-chain omega-3 was dramatically decreasing.

An estimated 90 to 95 percent decrease in fish oil consumption has taken place in the last one hundred years. Today the average American is now consuming 125 mg of long-chain omega-3 fatty acids from fish oil—while consuming approximately 20 grams per day of omega-6 fatty acids coming from cheap vegetable oils.

Once the last nutritional barrier (fish oil rich in omega-3 fatty acids) to prevent a rapid rise in inflammation was removed, all the pieces to generate the Perfect Nutritional Storm were in place to create the current epidemic of Toxic Fat Syndrome in the United States.

The first sign of this diet-induced inflammation that started twenty-five years ago was the rapid rise of obesity and its fellow traveler, type 2 diabetes. These two diseases have become epidemic in America and are now spreading throughout the world. To understand why, it helps to understand the complex nature of inflammation.

CHAPTER 3

How Inflammation Helps Us—and Hurts Us

W E OFTEN THINK OF INFLAMMATION IN TERMS OF PAIN, SOME-
thing to be avoided. But inflammation is one of the things
that keeps us alive in a hostile world. We live in a world
populated by microbial invaders, such as bacteria, fungi, parasites, and
viruses. Our internal inflammatory responses let us attack these invaders,
surround them, and ultimately kill them before they kill us. Likewise, it
is the same inflammatory responses that allow us to heal our bodies
when we become injured. The damaged tissue is sealed off while initial
pro-inflammatory responses destroy the damaged tissue, followed by
equally powerful internal anti-inflammatory responses that shut off the
inflammatory attack and begin to rebuild the damaged tissue. Through
advances in molecular biology, it is now known that there is another
event that can turn on the inflammatory response: your diet.

Without an adequate level of inflammation when called upon, we would be sitting ducks. We would be at the mercy of microbial invaders or injuries that would never heal. The inflammatory responses we have developed over millions of years are meant to keep this immunological warfare localized and highly concentrated. This is why it hurts. However, if an invading microbial invader escapes into the bloodstream, your inflammatory response becomes like a blind boxer constantly throwing punches. Although these punches rarely hit the opponent, they leave a lot of collateral damage throughout as the body is essentially attacking itself. This is why before the advent of antibiotics, death rates from systemic microbial invasions were virtually 100 percent. Even today, the mortality rate due to systemic microbial infections (such as bacterial sepsis) still remains incredibly high.

The complexity of inflammation comes from its two diametrically opposed parts. The pro-inflammatory attack response is generated in response to external events (such as infection, injury, or diet) and is followed by a corresponding generation of an internal anti-inflammatory response embedded in our genes. It is this internal anti-inflammatory response that not only turns off the attack phase of inflammation but also generates the repair processes that lead to cellular rejuvenation.

Let me give you an example. When you cut your hand, initially there is pain, swelling, and redness as the body tries to control the extent of the injury and the resulting invasion of microbes. This is the pro-inflammatory response (attack phase) in which microbial invaders are sealed off in a battle zone where they are surrounded and destroyed. Within a few days, the hand has completely healed. It has been rejuvenated at the cellular level. This is the internal anti-inflammatory response (resolution phase of inflammation) that is part of our genetic code. It is this complex orchestration of pro-inflammatory (cellular destruction) and anti-inflammatory (cellular rejuvenation) responses that constitutes our immune system.

Defining Wellness

Our current health-care system is based on managing the symptoms of chronic disease. This might be keeping cholesterol levels, blood sugar levels, or blood pressure under control with drugs. This approach treats the symptoms of the particular disease but not the underlying cause. We can easily define chronic disease by its symptoms, but we don't have a good definition of wellness. Obviously, saying you don't have a chronic disease is very different from being well because it takes years, if not decades, for any chronic disease to finally develop. During this time a person is not ill enough to be considered sick, but is definitely not well. So to truly describe wellness, we need a new definition.

I believe wellness can be defined by how well you keep the powerful pro-inflammatory and anti-inflammatory responses balanced. What we perceive as inflammation may be either too much of a pro-inflammatory response or not enough of an anti-inflammatory response. In either case, you will be under constant inflammatory attack. If you are unable to turn off the attack phase of inflammation completely, the body remains under constant inflammatory attack, but at a lower level of intensity. This is the insidious nature of a pro-inflammatory diet that causes Toxic Fat Syndrome. The end result is that your body moves toward developing chronic diseases associated with increased inflammation, such as diabetes, heart disease, cancer, and Alzheimer's. On the other hand, if you follow an anti-inflammatory diet, the result would be an increase in the cellular rejuvenation that takes place during the anti-inflammatory phase of the overall inflammatory response. This provides you with the holy grail of molecular medicine—continued cellular regeneration at any age.

Silent Inflammation

We usually associate inflammation with pain. This pain comes from the collateral damage of immunological warfare at the cellular level as the body tries to sequester microbial invaders or contain the damage induced by injuries. This is why the ancient Greeks described inflammation as the "internal fire." The ancient Romans described it in terms of heat, pain, redness, and swelling. These terms used to describe inflammation two thousand years ago are essentially the same ones most physicians use to describe inflammation today—which suggests that our understanding of inflammation hasn't increased that much over the past two thousand years! This is what I call classic inflammation. It hurts, and that's why you go to a doctor.

What if you had inflammation with no associated pain? This silent inflammation is the most dangerous type of inflammation because you do nothing about it as it continues to attack your organs for years until enough accumulated damage occurs to produce a visible chronic disease. After years and even decades of constant attack by this low-intensity, silent inflammation, a wide variety of chronic conditions may appear. When enough organ damage occurs, it begins to hurt. Then you go to a doctor. But the best your physician can do is give you drugs to treat the symptoms of the chronic disease—nothing to treat the underlying cause. While this is great news for drug companies who now have a lifetime customer, it's not good for you because the underlying cause is still there: the constant presence of silent inflammation.

The Role of Diet in Silent Inflammation

Our immune system was designed to protect us from alien invaders or injury. However, as I said earlier, your diet can also activate inflammation. In a sense, making the wrong food choices (like excessive consumption of cheap carbohydrates and cheap vegetable oils that make inflammatory hormones) can fool the body into thinking that it is under microbial attack. The consequences will not be as extreme in the short term as a real microbial attack or injury (that is, screaming pain), but the end result of this constant generation of low-level inflammation that is below the perception of pain (silent inflammation) is the acceleration of the development of future chronic disease.

Silent inflammation actually may be a condition that comes primarily from the radical changes in diet that have occurred over the past twenty-five years (the Perfect Nutritional Storm). The common diseases of Western civilization (heart disease, obesity, type 2 diabetes, and so on) are probably due in large part to these dietary changes that have increased the levels of silent inflammation. This has altered the body's natural inflammatory environment, resulting in the acceleration of these chronic diseases.

Since no pain is associated with silent inflammation, how do you know if you have high levels of it? Remember that the driving force behind silent inflammation is the increased level of toxic fat that I described earlier. This means the only way to really tell is by the blood tests that I will describe later in the book. Of course, if you already have a chronic disease, then you can be fairly certain you have high levels of silent inflammation and have had it for some time.

You can't tell the levels of silent inflammation people have in their blood by simply looking at them, just like you can't tell someone's cholesterol levels by looking at them. But there are simple, subjective ways to suggest that you may have high levels of systemic silent inflammation. The background behind these subjective parameters will be explained in greater detail in chapter 7, but here is a quick summary.

Keep in mind that no single parameter will tell you, but if you answer yes to more than three of these questions, it is quite likely that you probably have high levels of silent inflammation. Here are the questions you want to ask yourself:

➤ Are you overweight?
➤ Are you taking a cholesterol-lowering drug?
➤ Are you groggy upon waking?
➤ Are you prone to stress?
➤ Are you constantly craving carbohydrates?
➤ Are you fatigued throughout the day?
➤ Are you especially hungry two hours after dinner?
➤ Are your fingernails brittle?

You can see by looking at these questions that many Americans will probably answer at least three of them affirmatively, indicating that they have silent inflammation. I have come to the same conclusion based on thousands of blood tests I have run in the past several years to measure Toxic Fat Syndrome. In other words, there's a lot of silent inflammation out there, and it's getting worse.

How Silent Inflammation Reduces Wellness

You can think of our movement from wellness to chronic disease as mediated by increasing levels of toxic fat in our stored body fat leaking into the bloodstream and resulting in Toxic Fat Syndrome:

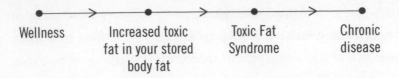

Wellness   Increased toxic   Toxic Fat   Chronic
fat in your stored   Syndrome   disease
body fat

This is why we sometimes make medicine too complex. If such a simple linkage between silent inflammation caused by Toxic Fat Syndrome, chronic disease, and wellness exists, then the magic elixir needed to maintain a state of wellness would simply be reducing silent inflammation in the body and keeping it under control for a lifetime.

Theoretically, we have a potential solution at hand—the lifetime use of anti-inflammatory drugs, which include aspirin, non-steroidal anti-inflammatories (such as Motrin), COX-2 inhibitors (Celebrex and Vioxx), and corticosteroids (prednisone). These drugs treat classic inflammation. Unfortunately, such a lifetime strategy to keep silent inflammation under control (which is itself a lifelong struggle) has significant possible drawbacks, including:

- ➤ Immune suppression
- ➤ Osteoporosis
- ➤ Heart attacks
- ➤ Heart failure
- ➤ Death

Of all these side effects that come with long-term use of anti-inflammatory drugs, it's the last side effect—death—that should get your attention. It is estimated that more people die each year in America from taking the correct dosage of anti-inflammatory drugs than die from AIDS. So using anti-inflammatory drugs on a lifetime basis is probably not the answer to treating silent inflammation and regaining your wellness. On the other hand, understanding how these drugs reduce standard inflammation provides the clue to how to achieve the same result by following an anti-inflammatory diet.

Eicosanoids

We know that all forms of inflammation (including silent inflammation) are ultimately controlled by a group of hormones known as eicosanoids (eye-ka-san-oids). The 1982 Nobel Prize was awarded to three researchers for their discoveries of the role eicosanoids play in the development of chronic disease.

It is the balance of eicosanoids in your body that is the ultimate key to wellness. Simply stated, the "good" eicosanoids promote cellular rejuvenation; the "bad" eicosanoids promote cellular destruction. You need both good and bad eicosanoids to survive. It's when the balance of these powerful hormones is disrupted and you start making too many bad eicosanoids that you begin moving away from wellness and toward the development of chronic disease.

This is where your diet enters the picture. All eicosanoids are ultimately derived from dietary fat, in particular the polyunsaturated essential fatty acids that must be supplied by the diet. There are only three such essential fatty acids that can be made into eicosanoids: dihomo-gamma-linolenic acid (DGLA), arachidonic acid (AA), and eicosapentaenoic acid (EPA).

DGLA and AA are omega-6 fatty acids, and EPA is an omega-3 fatty acid found in fish oil. The really good eicosanoids that accelerate cellular rejuvenation come from DGLA, the really bad eicosanoids that accelerate cellular destruction come from AA, and the eicosanoids that come from EPA don't do much. However, EPA does help maintain a dynamic balance between DGLA and AA as well as dilute out any excess AA in the cell. So in essence, your diet is the primary factor in keeping these three fatty acids constantly in balance. The better you do it, the less toxic fat you have, the more silent inflammation is reduced, and the faster you move back toward wellness.

That's why anti-inflammatory drugs have significant side effects (including death), because in the process of reducing bad eicosanoids, they also knock out the production of the good eicosanoids. The best example was Vioxx, the new wonder drug that could relieve pain without any side effects, so the drug manufacturer said. Unfortunately, Vioxx also knocked out the good ones that helped prevent heart attacks.

Trans fats also knock out the production of good eicosanoids because they decrease the production of dihomo-gamma-linolenic acid (DGLA). This is why there is a correlation between trans fats and heart disease. The next time you eat any processed food that uses partially hydrogenated vegetable oil as one of its ingredients, you might as well be taking a daily dose of Vioxx.

Food as a Drug

If the lifetime use of anti-inflammatory drugs isn't a good wellness strategy, are we doomed to the increasing appearance of chronic disease at a younger age? *Not if you are willing to change the way you eat.* As powerful as these eicosanoids are, they are completely under dietary control. An anti-inflammatory diet that decreases the bad eicosanoids while increasing the good eicosanoids will provide the dietary pathway to maintaining wellness simply by maintaining the optimal balance of both good and bad eicosanoids—not too high but not too low. This is why I developed the Zone Diet nearly twenty years ago. It is essentially a master dietary juggler that allows you to play this eicosanoid-balancing game with remarkable skill.

The Zone Diet: A Lifelong Anti-Inflammatory Diet

The Zone Diet is simply a way of life to keep the levels of silent inflammation under control for a lifetime by balancing a reduced glycemic load with the appropriate amount of protein at each meal coupled with the restriction of the omega-6 fatty acids. It's a lot easier than you think as I will discuss in chapter 8. You greatly enhance the anti-inflammatory actions of the Zone Diet by supplementing with adequate doses of fish oil (described in chapter 9). The combination of these two dietary interventions gives you a powerful dietary approach to greatly reduce silent inflammation and allow you to actually reverse the symptoms of chronic disease as you move back to a state of wellness.

That was my vision that started when the 1982 Nobel Prize was awarded for understanding the importance of eicosanoids in the development of chronic disease. At the time, I was doing research in intravenous cancer drug technology to reduce the inherent toxicity found in all cancer drugs. The goal in cancer chemotherapy is to keep the highly toxic cancer drug in a therapeutic zone. Too little of the drug, and the patient dies of cancer; too much and the patient dies from its toxic side effects. Using the appropriate drug delivery technologies, you could potentially reduce these toxicity problems and allow the cancer patient a chance to live a longer and better quality of life.

Because all eicosanoids are ultimately derived from dietary essential fatty acids, I reasoned that the secret to maintaining wellness was simply to induce the body to make more good eicosanoids and fewer bad ones. Without going much into the science (which is found in the back of the book in the appendices, thankfully, according to my wife), as toxic fat (AA) rises and DGLA decreases, you begin to lose wellness and begin the slow, steady descent toward chronic disease. The balance of these two fatty acids is dynamic, constantly changing with your diet. In particular, the level of insulin primarily controls this balance. If you eat too many high glycemic-load carbohydrates (bread, pasta, rice, and so on), insulin levels will increase. If you eat too few carbohydrates, cortisol levels will increase, and this will eventually also increase insulin levels. The Zone Diet keeps insulin in a healthy zone that is not too high, but not too low. This is why you can take an existing poor eicosanoid balance and rectify it *within 30 days.* But to keep that healthy eicosanoid balance, you will need to keep the hormonal responses generated by the diet "in the Zone" for a lifetime.

In simple terms, the balance of AA and DGLA will depend on your ability to control the balance of fat, protein, and carbohydrate that you eat. As AA levels increase, silent inflammation rises, and you age faster. On the other hand, if DGLA levels increase, you get more cellular rejuvenation, and you age more slowly. The ideal situation is to decrease AA levels while simultaneously increasing DGLA levels. If you do that, you essentially have the molecular definition of anti-aging, the lifelong maintenance of wellness.

The balance of AA and DGLA depends primarily on fat intake and, in particular, a precise balance of omega-6 and omega-3 fatty acids as well as the dietary balance of protein to carbohydrate to control the hormone insulin. The more omega-6 fatty acids in our diet, the more AA our bodies can ultimately produce. Although both DGLA and AA are omega-6 fatty acids, the hormone insulin is what accelerates the conversion of DGLA into AA. One way to increase insulin is to consume too many carbohydrates, especially refined carbohydrates. The second way is to eat too many calories. Americans have done both for the past twenty-five years due to the Perfect Nutritional Storm.

Toxic Fat Syndrome: The Spread of Silent Inflammation

Syndromes are clusters of symptoms that strongly predict future chronic disease if not corrected. Usually a syndrome has an underlying cause that manifests each of the symptoms. In many ways, a syndrome can be viewed as a balloon filled with water. If you push your hand on one side of this water-filled balloon, a protrusion will appear on the other side. Remove the pushing hand, and other side relaxes, and the balloon takes its natural shape once again. The pushing hand can be viewed as the underlying cause of the syndrome, and the protrusion on the other side as one, if not many, of the symptoms of the syndrome.

For example, metabolic syndrome is a cluster of symptoms, including being overweight, being shaped like an apple, having high triglycerides, and having low HDL cholesterol. The underlying cause of metabolic syndrome is elevated levels of insulin (hyperinsulinemia). While none of these symptoms of metabolic syndrome on its own is considered a disease, if all are present at the same time, then there is a very high likelihood of type 2 diabetes developing in eight to ten years if they are not corrected.

Toxic Fat Syndrome is no different. The underlying driving force for this syndrome is increased toxic fat in the bloodstream that is spreading silent inflammation throughout the bloodstream to attack the rest of the body. If chronic silent inflammation is left untreated, then the person has a very high likelihood of developing type 2 diabetes, heart disease, cancer, neurological disorders, asthma, allergies, auto-immune disorders, inflammatory diseases, and so forth. Both metabolic syndrome and Toxic Fat Syndrome can be compared to toxic shock syndrome as shown in the following chart.

Syndrome	Cause	Symptoms	Results if Untreated
Metabolic	Hyperinsulinemia	Abdominal obesity, high TG, low HDL	Development of type 2 diabetes in 8 to 10 years
Toxic Fat	Systemic spread of silent inflammation	Slow but relentless organ damage	Early development of chronic diseases
Toxic Shock	Hyperinflammation	Rapid organ failure caused by systemic bacterial invasion	Rapid organ failure and death

You can see from the chart that Toxic Fat Syndrome is not to be ignored.

Summary

Here is an easy summary of this chapter: *classic inflammation hurts; silent inflammation slowly kills.* Both types of inflammation are controlled by eicosanoids that can be manipulated by the diet for better or worse. One of the first signs of the presence of increasing levels of toxic fat in your body may be an increase in body fat (although thin people can have the problem as well). If the silent inflammation begins to spread into the bloodstream (Toxic Fat Syndrome), then other conditions, such as type 2 diabetes, heart disease, cancer, neurological disorders, and immunological disorders, will emerge much sooner than expected if Toxic Fat Syndrome is left unchecked.

CHAPTER 4

Why Getting Fat May Not Be Your Fault

Y OU DON'T HAVE TO BE A ROCKET SCIENTIST TO SEE THAT OBESITY is increasing in America. But why is it increasing? It depends on whom you talk to. Most people believe it is due to lack of self-control. They think people who are lean are simply morally superior to those who are fat; if fat people would only follow the standard refrain to "eat less and exercise more," obesity wouldn't be a problem.

I believe the underlying cause is far more complex. I am firmly convinced that the driving force behind obesity is *the growing level of silent inflammation induced by an increasingly pro-inflammatory diet.* As silent inflammation increases, it begins to disrupt hormonal signaling patterns, especially those that control appetite and how fat is released for energy. One of the first signs that silent inflammation is increasing is the appearance of excess body fat. Unless you reduce the levels of silent inflammation (especially in the fat cells), promoting simple political slogans to "eat less and exercise more" will never work in the long-term.

What Does a Calorie Actually Do?

Everyone talks about calories, but no one seems to be able to explain what they do. In reality, calories represent the amount of energy released when a food item is burned in a laboratory furnace. That is very different from what happens in the body, which converts incoming calories to chemical energy (known as adenosine triphosphate or ATP) that actually runs the body's metabolism. Calories are to ATP what crude oil is to gasoline. Without refining crude oil into gas, your car would never run. Likewise, without converting dietary calories into ATP, your body would never run.

Individual cells can store only about ten seconds' worth of ATP, so it must be made on demand on a second-by-second basis for you to stay alive. It's like stopping your car every hundred feet to refuel the gas tank. Fortunately, your body doesn't have to stop, because it can make more ATP from either stored carbohydrate or stored fat.

The body's ability to produce ATP from various components of the diet is highly variable. One gram of fat can make three times more ATP than one gram of carbohydrate. This is why I consider stored fat high-octane fuel, and stored carbohydrate low-octane fuel. Protein can't be used to make ATP unless it is broken down and reassembled into either carbohydrate or fat.

Regardless of the dietary source of calories, once the body has made enough ATP for its immediate energy needs, the vast majority of the remaining incoming calories, whatever their source, get converted into fat for long-term storage and eventual distribution to make more ATP at a later date.

Converting Excess Calories into Fat

The first step to store any excess macronutrient (protein, carbohydrate, or fat) for future use is turning that excess macronutrient into circulating fat (lipoproteins), which is done in the liver.

Of these three dietary macronutrients, the body has a limited ability to store excess carbohydrates and an even lesser ability to store excess dietary protein. If it could, then we could all look like Arnold Schwarzenegger by eating excess protein. But what the body can do very effectively is convert both excess carbohydrate and protein into fat, and that can be very easily stored in your fat cells.

Depending on the macronutrient, the efficiency of the conversion from what goes into your mouth into circulating fat in the bloodstream is highly variable. Obviously dietary fat requires the least amount of energy (about 3 percent of the calories in the dietary source of the fat) to absorb it and convert it into circulating fat carried by lipoproteins. Excess carbohydrates that can't be stored as glycogen (in the liver and muscles) require more energy (about 5 to 15 percent of their caloric energy) to be converted into circulating fat. Finally, excess protein has the least efficient conversion into circulating fat because it requires about 25 percent of the dietary calories to convert it into circulating fat. So you can quickly see that the type of macronutrient you are eating in excess has a great impact on the final levels of increased circulating fat.

The Fat Trap

The role of genetics is dominant in storing excess calories as fat. Some people store excess dietary calories as fat very easily; others store them with great difficulty. Studies with genetically modified animals confirm this, as do overeating studies in humans.

We eat in order to get sufficient calories to make enough ATP to run our bodies. If we don't, we either keep eating to get enough calories to make the necessary ATP, or we slow down all physical activity to conserve the limited amounts of ATP we have available from the calories we have consumed.

If you eat too much and are fat, you are considered a glutton. If you are fat and don't exercise a lot, you are considered a sloth. Often the two go together. But what if both are merely a secondary consequence of not being able to make enough ATP from incoming calories? The calories obviously went into your mouth. The fat trap is what happened to interrupt their flow into making ATP for your body.

In essence, the fat trap occurs in people who are genetically sensitive to insulin. For these individuals, excess incoming calories are converted to fat and enter the fat cells for storage. For many people, however, due to their genetic sensitivity to insulin, this stored fat will have great difficulty leaving the fat cells at a future time to make adequate ATP to fuel the body. If they try to "eat less and exercise more," they drive the body into a starvation mode with much less fat loss than would be predicted. Eating less decreases the amount of ATP the body can produce, while exercising more uses up the existing stores of ATP at a faster rate. They will lose weight, but much of that will come from their muscles and organs that are being cannibalized to make enough ATP to keep the body going as they "eat less and exercise more." What about the excess potential calories stored in their adipose tissue that could potentially make enough ATP to allow them to "eat less and exercise more"? As long as the fat trap is operating, these potential ATP-generating calories simply sit there.

The only way out of this fat trap is to decrease insulin levels by reducing carbohydrate intake. But this is a tricky game to play because if insulin levels are lowered too much by greatly restricting carbohydrates (as on the Atkins diet), the brain will not have enough glucose to make ATP for its energy needs. (Unlike other organs in your body, the brain can only use glucose for ATP production.) Your brain responds to decreased glucose levels in your bloodstream by increasing the production of the hormone cortisol, which breaks down muscle mass into glucose. Eventually the elevated cortisol levels make you fat again. The only way to overcome the fat trap on a long-term basis is to keep insulin levels in a zone that is not too high, but not too low.

That is the goal of the Zone Diet.

Understanding the Molecular Nature of the Fat Trap

Because the concept of "calories in equal calories out" is so ingrained in medical thinking, it is worth going into a little more detail about how the fat trap operates at the molecular level.

Remember, most excess calories we don't immediately use for ATP production will be converted into fat for storage. The only organ in the body that can safely store excess fat is adipose tissue. This is a massive collection of fat cells working together as a very sophisticated energy distribution system. Excess calories that enter our bodies as we eat are converted to fat in the liver where they are repackaged as lipoproteins. The lipoproteins deliver the fats to the surface of the fat cell where they are hydrolyzed to free fatty acids, then transported across the fat cell membrane by unique fatty acid binding proteins. The free fatty acids are immediately reassembled into triglycerides for safe, long-term storage in the adipose tissue. At some point in time, these stored fats are finally released back into the bloodstream to provide high-octane fuel to make adequate levels of ATP when the body needs it. When this distribution system runs efficiently, the fat in the adipose tissue is being rapidly turned over, with very little fat accumulation in the end.

The controller of this complex process is insulin. Every cell (including fat cells) has insulin receptors. Once insulin interacts with those receptors, a complex series of reactions occurs that removes excess glucose from the bloodstream and into the target cell.

In the fat cells, glucose gets converted into glycerol, which is needed in order to store any type of incoming free fatty acids. Without the adequate supply of free fatty acids or glycerol, it is hard for the fat cell to make new triglycerides that can be readily stored in them. In other words, it is difficult to become fat. The more insulin we have in the bloodstream, the more glucose is driven to the fat cells to make glycerol and the more fatty acid binding proteins are synthesized so that more free fatty acids can be transferred into the fat cells. The end result is your fat cells can store even more fat. This is why excess insulin makes us fat. Insulin also inhibits the release of this stored fat back into the circulation to make ATP. This is why excess insulin keeps us fat.

It is only when insulin levels fall, between meals or at night for instance, that the gate-keeping enzyme in the fat cell "relaxes" and lets stored fat begin to be released back into the bloodstream to supply raw material to the rest of the body to make the necessary ATP to keep you going.

If your fat cells are not genetically very sensitive to the release of stored fat by insulin, then the process of converting incoming calories to high-octane fuel (fat) and releasing them for further use works very smoothly. It's like a Wal-Mart warehouse. Goods from China are sent to the warehouse where they are stored for the short-term and then rapidly shipped out to the appropriate store. If the system is efficient, the warehouse never piles up with goods because distribution trucks are always being loaded and leaving the warehouse.

Here is where genetics come into play. If your fat cells are genetically sensitive to insulin, then incoming calories are still being converted to fat and being stored readily in the adipose tissue, but they are not leaving as quickly. It's as if the delivery trucks are no longer showing up at the Wal-Mart warehouse. You begin accumulating more and more stored fat in the adipose tissue. Many of your incoming dietary calories are simply being trapped in the fat cells—and the rest of the body becomes just as deficient in ATP production as if you had been starving yourself. Because this stored energy can't get out to the rest of the body to make enough ATP, you either keep eating more food (become a "glutton") or slow down any physical movement (become a "sloth") to conserve what limited ATP the rest of the body has to work with.

Energy Balance

So why don't people with a genetically determined fat trap continually increase in size like a balloon being filled up with air? Because stored fat never stops flowing completely from the fat cells back into the bloodstream, where it can be transported to other cells to be converted into ATP. This is known as energy homeostasis, a fancy phrase for energy balance. Enough of the incoming dietary calories that are not being trapped in adipose tissue escape so that the other organs in the body are able to make enough ATP for sustaining life. Once this balance is achieved, a weight plateau is established. This is true for both weight gain and weight loss in people with a fat trap.

Looking at weight gain from this perspective gives a radically new way to look at the obesity crisis. This is important since it is estimated that 75 percent of your ability to gain excess weight comes from your genes. You can't change your genes, but you can change whether those genes are turned on or turned off by your diet. This is why reducing the levels of insulin in the bloodstream can decrease the efficiency of a genetically determined fat trap. Unfortunately, the increased consumption of refined carbohydrates in the past twenty-five years has increased the efficiency of the fat trap in genetically susceptible individuals.

Treating obesity is solved not by "eating less and exercising more" but by reducing insulin levels generated by the diet so that more stored fat can be released for more ATP production. Only then can you eat less and exercise more without cannibalizing your muscles and organs. Obese individuals overeat (especially if their diet is high in carbohydrates) to ensure that enough ATP can be made to prevent them from starving. If they eat less, then they have fewer available calories that can be potentially converted into ATP. As a result, they start cannibalizing their muscles and organs in order to provide enough fuel to make ATP for the rest of the body. Just like any starving person, they will be obsessed with food. This is also the case in genetically obese animals. If their calorie intake is reduced, they will lose weight. But if you look at their organs upon autopsy, the fat stores are still immense (although slightly lower in size), but their organs and muscles are shriveled due to starvation.

Overeating for obese people is just their way around a genetically induced fat trap. Their overeating is not the primary cause of their obesity, but rather it is a secondary consequence of their genetics interacting adversely with excess insulin being produced by their diet. This prevents the release of high-octane fuel (fat) from the adipose tissue to make the necessary ATP that the rest of the body desperately needs to function.

Theoretically, the number of obese individuals should have remained fairly constant because genetics don't change that quickly. So what has happened in the last twenty-five years to cause the sudden rise in obesity? Americans are eating more carbohydrates. This increases insulin levels, which in turn increases the efficiency of their fat traps. Those who were genetically programmed to be overweight or obese are now becoming fatter.

What About Naturally Thin People?

The obese individual who overeats is considered a glutton. On the other hand, the normal-weight individual who overeats simply has a healthy appetite. The classic example is teenagers. Once they reach puberty, they are subjected to a surge of hormones that increase height, organ size, and muscle mass. All of these events require extraordinary amounts of ATP. The only way to achieve that is to eat extraordinary amounts of calories from any food item. After about age twenty, their maximum height and muscle mass have been achieved and their need for large increases in ATP decreases. If they don't start cutting back on calorie intake, then the excess calories no longer needed to fuel their growth are converted into fat. This becomes clearly obvious by age thirty as their clothes are not fitting the way they were at age twenty. They say their metabolism has changed. The reality is that their need for extra ATP production is no longer present.

However, there are some people who continue to be able to eat large amounts of calories and remain thin throughout their adult life. On closer inspection, this subgroup of people also has a different genetically induced metabolic problem compared to those who have a genetic predisposition for a fat trap. They are not very efficient in making ATP from incoming calories being released from the fat cells. They don't have a fat trap, but many of the fatty acids being released from the adipose tissue are being converted into excess free radicals instead of being converted into ATP. Going back to my Wal-Mart warehouse analogy, plenty of delivery trucks are taking the products out of the adipose tissue, but many of those products are falling off the truck before they ever reach the store.

Lean adults with inefficient metabolisms need to overeat to make sure they have enough excess calories to make enough ATP for the rest of their bodies' needs. Unfortunately for them, the excess free radicals being produced from their inefficient metabolism of fat are increasing their rate of aging. (I described this in one of my earlier books, *The Anti-Aging Zone*.)

Simple Thinking Doesn't Work

In both examples, the same behavior (overeating) results from the same underlying cause—the inability to make adequate levels of ATP for the body to run itself. In one case, the obese individual has a genetic sensitivity to insulin that inhibits the efficient release of stored fat that is necessary to make ATP. In the other case, the lean individual who overeats is very inefficient in metabolizing released fat into ATP. Both try to resolve their genetic problems by eating more calories until they can finally make enough ATP for the body.

This is why the simple thinking that eating less is the key to treating obesity is dead wrong. It's wrong because it is based on an equation that states:

*"Calories in must **equal** calories out."*

This equation is simply not valid because it doesn't reflect the reality of metabolism. The true equation that governs metabolism is this:

*"Incoming calories that can be easily converted to ATP must **equal** the amount of ATP required to keep the body going and to move around."*

If you reduce the body's ability to make ATP from incoming calories (either due to an efficient fat trap or inefficient ATP production), you have to either (1) eat more, (2) slow down physical activity, or (3) start cannibalizing your muscles and organs to get those extra calories to make the necessary amounts of ATP. This is why those obese individuals genetically predisposed to have a very efficient fat trap, as well as the lean person with a "healthy appetite," will always be starving when they start eating fewer calories. They can't change their genes, but the good news is they *can* alter the expression of those genes.

The person with a fat trap has to constantly keep levels of insulin low enough to reduce the inhibition on the release of stored body fat to make adequate levels of ATP, but not so low that blood glucose drops to the point that the brain doesn't have enough energy to make ATP. In other words, you have to keep insulin in a zone. Following the Zone Diet as described in chapter 8 can accomplish both tasks. The overweight and obese individuals can overcome their genetic predisposition for having a fat trap by following the Zone Diet, which keeps insulin levels as low as possible without compromising other functions of insulin (like driving nutrients into cells). The person with an inefficient metabolism should also follow the Zone Diet to generate the maximum amount of ATP with the least number of calories and therefore reduce excessive free radical generation. These are two different metabolic problems, but they have one dietary solution.

Why We Overeat

Understanding how the adipose tissue can trap incoming calories into long-term fat storage is only one-half of the story of how we get fat. The other part is why we have been overeating during the past twenty-five years. I don't believe it's due to better food marketing, but rather it is caused by hormonal changes induced by increased levels of toxic fat in the brain.

For all the talk about overeating, we still know surprisingly very little about it at the molecular level. (See appendix C for more details.) What we do know is there are two powerful biological urges that must be balanced if we are going to maintain an ideal weight. One is hunger; the other is satiety or lack of hunger. If these urges are balanced, then permanent weight control is easy.

Biological urges are not controlled by willpower. Try holding your breath to see how much willpower can prolong your ability not to breathe. Hunger is another such biological urge not easily handled by willpower. Obviously, if hunger is greater than satiety, the end result is weight gain, especially if food is readily accessible. A wide number of hormones control both hunger and satiety, and in particular, many of these hormones can be directly altered by the food you eat. This is why hormonal responses to macronutrients in the diet (carbohydrate, protein, and fat) can either accelerate hunger or reduce it. In particular, it is excess carbohydrates that are the primary culprit in generating hunger, whereas protein is the prime player in generating satiety.

Hunger

Not surprisingly, most of the control of hunger and satiety is located in the brain, in the hypothalamus to be precise. Much of hunger is driven by the brain's need for a constant supply of glucose for ATP production. (Glucose is the primary fuel source for ATP production for the brain.) When blood glucose levels drop in the brain, it goes into a panic mode in an effort to get more glucose into the bloodstream for it to extract for its own ATP production. The easiest solution is to eat more calories, especially those rich in carbohydrates that can be converted rapidly into glucose. This means grains and starches, and especially processed foods composed of refined carbohydrates coming from grains and starches. The faster the glucose enters the bloodstream, the quicker it gets to the brain to quell its immediate need for ATP production.

The same rapid increase in blood glucose causes the pancreas to release more insulin that will drive blood sugar levels lower again within a few hours so you are hungry again. The end result is constant hunger even in the face of excess calorie consumption. Think of eating a big bowl of pasta at noon, and then being hungry two hours later. And where do excess calories end up, especially in the presence of excess insulin? As stored fat.

Unfortunately, you don't have to eat too many excess carbohydrates to cause insulin levels to begin to increase in the bloodstream. Even worse is if you develop a condition known as insulin resistance where insulin levels are constantly elevated even in the absence of carbohydrates. This occurs when the insulin receptor in the muscle cells becomes desensitized. As a result, the pancreas begins to secrete greater amounts of insulin into the blood to overcome this resistance, to try to bring blood glucose levels under control. (High levels of blood glucose can be toxic.) If you have insulin resistance, then your fat trap will become even more activated, making even less fat available for ATP production. You respond by eating more calories, especially carbohydrates rich in glucose (grains and starches) that drive up insulin levels, and the cycle continues. Not only does excess insulin make you fat and keep you fat, but it also makes you continuously hungry.

Another group of recently discovered hormones also increases hunger. These are called endocannabinoids. Although these hormones have been around for hundreds of millions of years, our knowledge of them only started with the greater use of marijuana in the 1960s.

One of the most common experiences of anyone who has ever smoked marijuana is a dramatically increased appetite (the "munchies"). The isolated active ingredient of marijuana is called tetrahydrocannabinol or THC. Researchers soon found that THC binds to certain receptors in the brain. Because these receptors existed for some other purpose than waiting for a person's first encounter with marijuana, it was hypothesized that something in the brain naturally binds to the same receptors to also cause ravenous hunger. These hypothetical hormones were named endocannabinoids. It was only years later that these hormones were isolated and found to be derived from toxic fat (arachidonic acid).

So the more arachidonic acid you have in the brain, the more endocannabinoids you have to stimulate hunger. Unfortunately, one consequence of the Perfect Nutritional Storm is its impact on increased arachidonic acid formation. This ensured that many people would soon have a lot more endocannabinoids in their brains, and therefore have a lot more hunger on their minds.

Two other hormones make you hungry. One is neuropeptide Y (NPY). When NPY is elevated in the brain, animals will literally eat themselves to death. The other is ghrelin, which comes from the gut, telling the brain there are no calories down there so it should start thinking about eating again. As I will discuss shortly, both of these hormones can also be controlled by the diet.

Satiety

Satiety is simply the lack of hunger between meals. If you aren't hungry, then cutting back on calories is very easy. On the other hand, if you are always hungry, then cutting back on calories requires constant willpower (think of holding your breath). The primary dietary factor in satiety is protein consumption, for two reasons. The first is that dietary protein increases the production of glucagon, a hormone with the opposite effect of insulin. Glucagon increases blood sugar (by mobilizing stored carbohydrates in the liver) rather than reducing blood sugar as insulin does. Simply stated, if the brain is getting adequate levels of glucose for ATP production, then it's happy and you aren't hungry. On the other hand, if the brain isn't getting adequate levels of glucose, you will be constantly hungry.

The second reason is that protein also has the additional benefit of releasing another recently discovered hormone, peptide YY (PYY), from the gut that travels directly to the brain to shut down hunger. It is the combination of both these hormones (glucagon and PYY) generated by dietary protein that produces much of the satiety response. Because PYY is released from the gut, it has the ability to inhibit the hunger signals generated by ghrelin. It makes a very nice "on-off" switch to tell the brain what is happening in the gut.

Another key hormone is leptin, which is released from your fat cells to travel to the brain to signal satiety because your fat stores are sufficient. In a perfect world, the more fat cells you have, the more leptin you generate, and once the brain receives leptin's signal, it should cause you to stop eating. Unfortunately, we don't live in a perfect world, and some people develop leptin resistance, which is similar to insulin resistance. The result is that leptin never reaches the brain in sufficient levels to signal satiety even though you have excess body fat. The underlying cause of both insulin and leptin resistance is increased silent inflammation. It has been shown that obese people have much higher levels of leptin in the blood, but they are constantly hungry—because if you have leptin resistance and not enough leptin is getting through, the brain tells you to keep eating.

Ironically, insulin can also function as a satiety hormone if it can get into the brain. Once in the brain, it will inhibit the release of NPY (the powerful hunger hormone mentioned earlier). If enough insulin is unable to get into the brain, then NPY is continually generated, and you are always hungry. This is another reason you don't want insulin levels to become too low.

The balancing precision of these hormone systems that control hunger and satiety is remarkable. If there is more than a 0.01 percent difference (a little more than 10 calories per day) between this constant battle of hunger and satiety, you can potentially gain about one pound of fat per year. Should the difference increase to about 0.1 percent (a little more than 100 calories per day), you can potentially gain ten pounds of fat on a yearly basis. For the past twenty-five years, we have been eating more because we have been hungrier. For females, this increase in calorie consumption has been about 350 calories per day, and for males it has been about 150 calories per day, and most of those increased calories have come from refined carbohydrates that stimulate insulin.

Why We Are Getting Fatter

Not everyone in America is getting fatter at the same rate. Those who are already overweight and obese are accounting for the rapid increase in obesity. These are the same people with a genetic predisposition for their adipose tissue to act as a fat trap. The increase in carbohydrate consumption over the past twenty-five years has led to an increase in their insulin levels. This increase in diet-induced insulin coupled with increasing insulin resistance has made the fat traps in these genetically susceptible people even more effective—ensuring that more and more of the extra incoming calories they are eating are being trapped in the adipose tissue. The end result is the fat are getting fatter.

At the same time, we have been becoming hungrier. This is related to the combined impact of increased insulin on decreasing blood sugar levels as well as the increase of endocannabinoids in the brain due to increased levels of toxic fat.

All of this can be traced back to the advent of the Perfect Nutritional Storm and its impact on increasing silent inflammation.

Inflammation and Obesity

It has always been known that inflammation and obesity seem to occur together. The question is, "Does obesity cause inflammation, or does inflammation cause obesity?"

One way to find answers is to hold a conference, and that's what

Harvard Medical School did in March 2007. The studies presented at that conference gave strong evidence that inflammation precedes obesity. As one of the speakers, Eric Rimm, associate professor of epidemiology and nutrition at Harvard Medical School, said, "We don't have an obesity epidemic; we have an inflammation epidemic."

So how could increased inflammation become the primary factor behind the obesity crisis? To understand the answer, we need to look at the production of toxic fat (arachidonic acid, known as AA), and how the Perfect Nutritional Storm has increased its levels in the body.

The body needs some AA, but too much can have significant adverse health consequences (such as death). Two dietary factors have worked to keep AA from becoming too elevated in humans: the balance of omega-6 fatty acids and omega-3 fatty acids, and the balance of protein to carbohydrate in the diet. Both of these factors interact with the key enzyme (delta-5-desaturase) that produces AA.

Like most key enzymes in the body, this enzyme is controlled primarily by hormones, specifically insulin and glucagon, as well as the omega-3 fatty acid known as eicosapentaenoic acid (EPA) as shown in the following diagram.

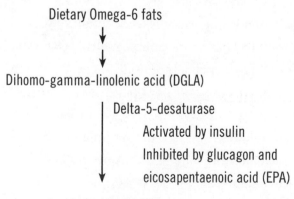

Dietary Omega-6 fats

↓
↓

Dihomo-gamma-linolenic acid (DGLA)

Delta-5-desaturase
Activated by insulin
Inhibited by glucagon and
eicosapentaenoic acid (EPA)

Arachidonic acid (AA)

Dihomo-gamma-linolenic acid (DGLA) is the building block of the good eicosanoids that rejuvenate cells, whereas arachidonic acid (AA) is the building block of the bad eicosanoids that put the immune system constantly into an attack mode, thus causing cellular destruction.

Until the 1920s, excess omega-6 fatty acids were relatively rare in the American diet because our major sources of dietary fat were pork lard, butter, and fish oil. These have been replaced by cheap vegetable oils (corn, soy, sunflower, and safflower) that are rich in omega-6 fatty acids. As the levels of omega-6 fatty acids are increased in the diet, we increase the likelihood of producing more AA. It's like adding more water to a water tower: The pressure at the bottom gets greater and greater. At the same time, the levels of long-chain omega-3 fatty acids coming from fish oil have dramatically decreased. In particular, high levels of EPA are needed to partly inhibit the activity of the delta-5-desaturase enzyme. This sudden shift in the balance of these fatty acids in the American diet has dramatically increased the production of arachidonic acid, thus increasing silent inflammation.

What has made a bad situation worse is the simultaneous increase in insulin production caused by the increased consumption of processed foods rich in refined carbohydrates, including pasta, pizza, and bread. In the past twenty-five years, the levels of carbohydrates (especially refined carbohydrates) have been climbing in the American diet. These refined carbohydrates are virtually pure glucose, and when they enter the bloodstream, production of the hormone insulin increases, which in turn activates the delta-5-desaturase enzyme to make even more AA (toxic fat).

This is why mixing excess omega-6 fatty acids (coupled with decreased EPA consumption) with excess insulin is like adding gasoline to a fire. The end result is more AA, which means more silent inflammation. With that increased silent inflammation comes its fellow travelers, insulin (and leptin) resistance. Couple this with increased endocannabinoids in the brain to generate constant hunger, and you get an obesity epidemic.

Complex Problems Aren't Solved by Simple Thinking

One simplistic answer in the past to the obesity crisis was, "If no fat touches my lips, then no fat will reach my hips." Because dietary fat requires the least amount of energy to be converted into circulating fat, then common sense would dictate that removing as much fat from the diet as possible would solve the obesity crisis. The problem is that dietary fat has no impact on insulin, and it is excess insulin that makes you fat and keeps you fat. This is also why it is impossible for dietary fat alone to make you fat. In fact, if you feed people a diet of pure fat, they would start losing weight (especially stored fat) because it is elevated insulin that prevents the release of stored fat. Of course, if you ate only fat, both the brain (which needs carbohydrates) as well as your muscles, the synthesis of new enzymes and other structural proteins, and your immune system (which all need a constant supply of protein) would suffer dire consequences.

Likewise, stating "a calorie is a calorie" is equally simplistic and misleading. Remember, the number of calories coming in that can be converted to useful ATP production has to equal the amount of ATP expended to keep us alive and to maintain a stable body weight. If many of those incoming dietary calories are trapped in the adipose tissue, then we have to either eat more calories or move around less to make the equation hold. Futhermore, the hormonal effect of a calorie of carbohydrate (which stimulates insulin) is different than a calorie of protein

45

(which stimulates glucagon and PYY), which is still different than a calorie of fat (which stimulates eicosanoids—both good and bad).

Finally, that overused slogan "eat less and exercise more" also tends to fail because no one had ever thought of the consequences of this dietary strategy on ATP production in individuals with genetic predisposition for a fat trap. Nowhere is that more evident than in childhood obesity. Two different large-scale studies (one in 1999 and the other in 2003), long-term and placebo-controlled (and very expensive), have been done with thousands of children, teaching them to eat less and exercise more. The end result was that the children became much more knowledgeable about nutrition and exercised more, but it had little impact on their weight. The apparent answer of the research community to these negative published trials? Let's pretend such studies don't exist and keep telling our children to eat less and exercise more. In the middle of the Perfect Nutritional Storm, that strategy is doomed to failure.

The Heaviest Man in the World

What happens when you begin to reduce insulin levels and rebalance hunger and satiety by reversing the hormonal consequences of the Perfect Nutritional Storm? One of the best examples is Manuel Uribe of Monterrey, Mexico. In early 2006, Manuel weighed more than 1,200 pounds and had not left his bed for more than five years. When my Mexican colleagues Gustavo and Silvia Orozco told him that they believed appropriate dietary changes could be his solution, his first response was, "You have to be kidding." After all, he had tried every diet known to mankind for the past five years and had only ended up gaining more weight. But the Orozcos were persistent because their secret weapon included high-dose fish oil to reduce endocannabinoids (the hormones in the brain that cause hunger) and to reduce the silent inflammation in his fat cells, as well as the Zone Diet to reduce insulin levels. Within a matter of days, Manuel was no longer hungry and was losing weight for the first time in five years. In fact, his major complaint was that he couldn't eat all the food he was supposed to (about 2,000 calories per day). In the first eighteen months, he lost more than 300 pounds, but the most exciting part was the changes in his blood chemistry. His cholesterol is normal (190 mg/dl), his HDL cholesterol is normal (55 mg/dl), his triglycerides are low (45 mg/dl), his blood sugar is normal (88 mg/dl), and his insulin levels are normal (10 uU/ml). In addition, his resting heart rate has dropped to 62 beats per minute, a level usually found in trained athletes, and his blood pressure is 120/70 (typical of a teenager). At the time of writing this book, Manuel has lost another 140 pounds, and his blood chemistry is even better. Manuel may be one of the healthiest men in Mexico even though he still weighs a little less than 800 pounds.

Manuel continues to lose weight because he is never hungry. The reason is the combination of the Zone Diet (to reduce insulin levels in the blood) and high-dose fish oil (to reduce endocannabinoid levels in the brain). It will take him another four years to get to his goal weight of 220 pounds. In reality, Manuel is already eating as if he weighs 220 pounds and is still having trouble eating all the food. I am confident he will be successful because he has a clinically proven pathway to balance the hormones that control hunger and satiety as well as allow him to tap into his fat stores to make all the ATP his body requires.

Summary

The Perfect Nutritional Storm has been the underlying cause of a radical change in the balance of diet-generated hormones in our bodies for the past twenty-five years. The result is increasing hunger as well as increasing the likelihood for those with existing genetic predispositions to increasingly store incoming calories in a fat trap. If you want permanent weight control, you must keep those hormones that control fat accumulation and the balance of hunger and satiety in the brain in a zone that is not too high, but not too low. You can do this by eating the appropriate balance of protein, carbohydrate, and fat that is right for your genetics. You just have to do it for a lifetime.

CHAPTER 5

Good Fat May Be Protective

EVEN THOUGH ONE OF THE FIRST INDICATIONS OF THE PRESENCE of increased silent inflammation is increased body fat accumulation, initially this excess fat may be protective. How can excess fat possibly be good? It can act as a powerful regulatory mechanism to control the malignant spread of toxic fat, thus preventing the development of Toxic Fat Syndrome. As a result, some excess fat may be a key to your longevity under the right circumstances.

Good Fat

The definition of good fat is a vast collection of healthy fats. Unlike any other cell in the body, a healthy fat cell can expand to encapsulate incoming excess calories that have been converted to fat as discussed in the last chapter. This is a great survival benefit in times of famine as it ensures that you will have plenty of raw material to make enough adenosine triphosphate (ATP) until the famine is over. Unfortunately, in America we define famine as more than two hours between snacks.

We rarely think about fat as an organ, like the heart or liver, but it is. The organ that stores your fat is the adipose tissue. For years it was thought that the adipose tissue was simply a storage site for fat. Now we know that it is a very complex organ that is in constant hormonal communication with every other organ, including the brain. The adipose tissue also has a very special trait—it can grow new fat cells with relative ease. Other organs, like the brain and muscle, can only do this with great difficulty, if at all. In the presence of the appropriate hormonal signals, the adipose tissue—which is rich in stem cells—will readily make new fat cells from these stem cells that can accommodate even greater levels of stored fat.

This ability to create new healthy fat cells is a very ingenious way to address two potential problems that would otherwise reduce your longevity:

- Preventing fat from being stored in all the wrong places (lipotoxicity)
- Providing a toxic waste dump to sequester fat-soluble toxins (including toxic fat) and to prevent them from attacking other organs

Preventing Lipotoxicity

Only one organ in the body is designed to contain a lot of fat: adipose tissue. The ability to store excess fat in adipose tissue prevents fat from going to all the wrong places. Fat compromises the function of other organs where it is deposited, leading to early chronic disease.

The most extreme example of this is a condition known as *lipodystrophy*, in which a person actually has no fat cells. Although you might think people with this condition would look great in swimsuits, in reality they more closely resemble Porky Pig. This is because with no adipose tissue to safely store fat, it spreads to all the wrong places—excess fat gets stored as lipid droplets in other organs. And with that type of fat comes a boatload of trouble. Whether in the liver, the muscles, the heart, or the pancreas, this excess fat accumulation in these cells compromises their primary functions. This is called lipotoxicity, and it leads to the rapid development of type 2 diabetes and heart disease as well as a fatty liver. Fortunately, for most of us with healthy fat cells, the adipose tissue comes to the rescue by essentially sucking up any excess fat that we eat or is produced by the body and storing it in an organ where it can't cause any damage. In essence, adipose tissue acts as a fat-buffering system, which can readily expand to protect you from your own dietary habits and prevent lipotoxicity that will shorten your life.

Excess Fat as a Toxic Waste Dump

The second great benefit of excess fat is that it is a great toxic waste dump for fat-soluble toxins. We are now exposed daily to a frightening new array of synthetic chemicals (such as herbicides, pesticides, PCBs, dioxins, flame retardants, plasticizers, and so forth) that have appeared only in the last seventy years, and many of these chemicals are fat-soluble. Good thing, too, because your adipose tissue can sequester these fat-soluble toxic chemicals and keep them in deep storage away from the rest of your body. The fatter you are, the greater the capacity to store these very toxic fat-soluble chemicals out of harm's way.

One of the most toxic fat-soluble chemicals is the natural fatty acid that has been around for hundreds of millions of years. This is arachidonic acid (AA), which in high enough concentrations can kill. This is why it can be considered toxic fat. It slowly kills by increasing silent inflammation, which is the driving force behind the development of virtually every chronic disease.

Remember, the body needs some AA to make enough pro-inflammatory eicosanoids to launch an appropriate immunological attack to repel alien invaders, such as bacteria, fungi, parasites, and viruses. However, if you make too much AA, it can turn on you, causing the immune system to be constantly turned on. Now your own immune system begins attacking every one of your organs slowly, but relentlessly.

The body goes to great lengths to maintain just enough AA in each of its 100 trillion cells. Any extra AA that is made or ingested gets sent to the adipose tissue for long-term storage, just like burying toxic nuclear waste. In this way, excess fat is acting like a buffering system for excess AA, keeping the levels of silent inflammation low in other body organs. Paradoxically, this is why fat accumulation (although one of the first signs of increasing silent inflammation) may initially be protective.

However, excess AA in any one cell (even the fat cells) can also be toxic. An ingenious way to overcome this problem is to get the adipose tissue to make more fat cells to help dilute the levels of AA in other fat cells before it causes an otherwise healthy fat cell to become sick and eventually die. It turns out that certain eicosanoids derived from AA do exactly that.

These eicosanoids derived from AA stimulate the stem cells in the adipose tissue to make new fat cells. It may be this ancient mechanism is an internal protective mechanism that didn't need to be widely invoked until the rise of diet-induced silent inflammation that began twenty-five years ago. That increase in silent inflammation was accompanied by such a dramatic increase in obesity that it can't be explained by the usual suspects of sloth and gluttony. Even though increased AA will cause the proliferation of new fat cells in the adipose tissue, these newly formed fat cells provide an increased toxic waste capacity to suck up any additional AA from the bloodstream. This prevents systemic inflammatory attacks on other organs. (That's a good thing.)

Basically, the less toxic fat you have floating in the bloodstream, the longer you are going to live, regardless of your weight. As far as the body is concerned, it is far better to be fat and not inflamed than to be a normal weight and inflamed. It's the silent inflammation that kills, not the excess weight.

"A Very Puzzling Disconnect"

We want to believe that normal-weight people live longer than overweight or obese individuals. Unfortunately, data from the Centers for Disease Control (CDC) show otherwise. The authors of this study, published in 2005, looked at the relationship of mortality to body mass index or BMI. BMI is simply a crude formula based on the height and weight that places you into different classifications:

BMI Classification	
Less than 18.5	Underweight
18.5 to 25	Normal weight
25 to 30	Overweight
30 to 35	Obese
35 to 40	Severely obese
Greater than 40	Morbidly obese

When the CDC analyzed mortality statistics for large populations, it was found that overweight people lived longer than normal-weight individuals, and that the mortality of even obese (BMI 30 to 35) individuals was not that much greater than those with normal weight. Yes, at the extremes of severe and morbid obesity, as well as the underweight, mortality increases. But in the middle, between normal weight, overweight, and non-severely obese, the death rate was about the same (and actually the lowest in the overweight category). An even larger 2006 study from the Mayo Clinic demonstrated that overweight people have a lower risk of not only overall mortality but also less cardiovascular mortality. Even obese subjects had no greater risk of either total or cardiovascular mortality than normal-weight subjects. In 2007, the CDC published a more complete report that showed that for some diseases, such as pneumonia, infections, or injuries, there was a nearly 40 percent reduction in mortality in overweight individuals compared to normal-weight individuals.

Talk about making the medical establishment mad. Here are two of their own rocking the foundation of our public health-care programs to make everyone in America normal weight. As JoAnn Mason, chief of preventive medicine at Harvard's Brigham and Women's Hospital, stated, "This is a very puzzling disconnect."

However, the explanation of this paradox is actually quite simple: the overweight individuals had more good fat to encapsulate any excess toxic fat than normal-weight individuals did.

There is no doubt that there is a correlation between excess body fat and many chronic diseases. This is why many have automatically assumed that excess weight is the actual cause of diseases such as heart disease, diabetes, cancer, Alzheimer's, and so forth. However, it is not excess weight, but *the spread of silent inflammation into the bloodstream.*

Therefore, if you are overweight or even obese but don't have Toxic Fat Syndrome, you may be healthy now, but all that could change any day. However, if you are fat *and* have Toxic Fat Syndrome, your future is not too bright.

The existence of good fat (that is, healthy fat cells) that can encapsulate any excess AA begins to explain the otherwise confusing data that overweight people outlive normal-weight individuals.

Metabolically Healthy Obese

Disease is defined as any condition that disrupts normal body function. By this definition, obesity *per se* is not a disease any more than being tall is. This is why a surprising number of obese individuals seem to be relatively healthy. These people are normal in every aspect except for the amount of excess fat they carry on their bodies.

They are called the metabolically healthy obese. This is not to say that accumulation of excess body fat is not a major concern, but the real question we should be asking is whether or not these excess levels of fat are leading to increased silent inflammation in other organs. For example, a 2005 study from Italy indicates that nearly 30 percent of morbidly obese Italians (average BMI of 40) are considered to be extremely healthy despite their obesity classification. Likewise, a 2004 study of morbidly obese Chinese patients (BMI greater than 40) going in for gastric bypass surgery revealed that nearly 50 percent had perfectly normal lipid levels. In other words, many of these obese Italians and Chinese were definitely fat but apparently healthy. They were sequestering excess toxic fat in their adipose tissue.

If excess toxic fat is confined to adipose tissue, little organ damage occurs outside the adipose tissue because the potentially damaging excess toxic fat is encapsulated. In fact, the continued growth of your adipose tissue may be your best initial defense to prevent the systematic spread of excess toxic fat to other tissues.

As long as the body can continue to sequester more and more of the AA being produced by the diet in its fat cells, the body fat will play the role of a benign adipose tumor that is protective—at least for now. However, should the fat cells in the adipose tissue become sick and eventually die due to excess AA accumulation, this begins a cascade of molecular events that eventually results in the rapid leakage of the stored excess AA into the bloodstream. Once it is there, it can begin to spread toxic fat to other organs, causing widespread inflammatory damage and potentially early cellular death in other organs such as the heart and brain. Unfortunately, these organs do not have the regenerative capacity of fat cells. So as more cells die in other organs, overall organ function is decreased. That's what you call chronic disease.

Good Fat in Children?

In fact, the continued growth of your adipose tissue may be the best initial defense to prevent the systematic spread of excess AA to other tissues even at an early age. This is illustrated in a 2000 study of 475 children in Crete who had perfectly normal lipid levels. However, if you look at the levels of AA in their adipose tissue, a very different picture emerges. The more overweight the child, the higher the levels of AA in the adipose tissue. What this suggests is that as the levels of AA rise in the body, an adaptation occurs to increase the amount of adipose tissue to keep the ever-increasing levels of AA sequestered from the rest of the body.

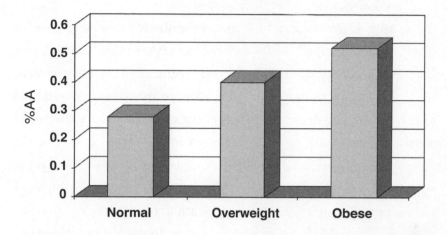

AA in Adipose Tissue
Increases with Weight

For these children in Crete, increasing amounts of excess fat were acting as a protective mechanism to sequester more and more of the AA being produced by their diets.

Unfortunately in America, we don't have the same situation. Virtually every obese child whom I have tested has high levels of Toxic Fat Syndrome. This means that the levees of their toxic waste dump have been breached, and toxic fat is now spilling into the bloodstream. Their future is not so bright.

Why Extra Fat Can Be Protective—at First

Let me make one thing clear: I am not advocating that people should begin getting fatter in hopes of improving their longevity. If that stored AA in the fat cells is released into the bloodstream, then all the chronic diseases associated with Toxic Fat Syndrome (type 2 diabetes, heart disease, cancer, neurological disorders, and so on) begin to emerge at a much earlier age. But not everyone who is overweight or even obese becomes diabetic, has heart disease, or develops cancer. As long as the excess AA is contained in the adipose tissue, the rest of your organs are spared from a constant inflammatory attack by the pro-inflammatory eicosanoids derived from it. On the other hand, if AA is being released from its toxic waste dump (adipose tissue), it can spread inflammation to every other organ, and you will see a very close association between obesity and mortality.

Summary

Deeply imbedded in our genes are mechanisms that may have only been recently activated by the growing epidemic of toxic fat. In essence, with recent inflammatory changes in our diet, we may be better off being overweight or even obese as it *can* protect you from Toxic Fat Syndrome. Yet we know that obesity is associated with increased diabetes and heart disease. These conflicting observations become reconciled once you understand how good fat (healthy fat cells) initially protects you from Toxic Fat Syndrome. Unfortunately, as the levels of toxic fat continue to increase in your fat cells, the risk of it spreading into your bloodstream and causing Toxic Fat Syndrome greatly increases. When this happens, you have malignant toxic fat.

CHAPTER 6

Malignant Toxic Fat

A FTER READING THE LAST CHAPTER, YOU MAY BE CONGRATULATING yourself on your extra stored body fat. Don't. While extra body fat may initially be protective, it can also turn on you at any time.

Here are some additional paradoxes about extra body fat. If extra fat can be protective by encapsulating excess arachidonic acid (AA), then how can it be associated with so many chronic disease conditions? And why are some overweight and even obese people actually very healthy? To make the connection between excess body fat, the loss of wellness, and the eventual development of chronic disease, you have to look at obesity from a radical new perspective: you have to start thinking of excess body fat as an adipose tumor, just like cancer in any other organ.

The real problem starts when stored toxic fat (AA) in the adipose tissue becomes malignant.

It is ironic that after spending much of my early research career developing drug delivery systems to treat cancer, I have come full circle to understand obesity as a tumor, in particular a tumor of the adipose tissue. Only by thinking outside the box of the traditional nutritional paradigms can many of the seeming inconsistencies of the global obesity epidemic be explained. More important, this way of thinking about obesity provides a revolutionary new approach to reverse the obesity epidemic caused by silent inflammation as well as the chronic disease conditions associated with Toxic Fat Syndrome.

When you begin to think of obesity as a tumor, you begin to notice a number of similarities between obesity and classic cancers:

➤ Localized uncontrolled tumor growth
➤ Significant inflammation in the primary tumor site
➤ Tumors that can be benign or malignant
➤ Patient is never "cured"

One of the great fallacies about both obesity and cancer is that you can be cured. The reason you got the cancer or developed obesity is that you are genetically predisposed, and under the right environmental conditions (that is, increased silent inflammation) both conditions can emerge. You can't change your genes, but you can change the expression of those genes through your diet. But make no mistake about it—you are looking at a lifelong commitment.

To protect yourself from high levels of systemic silent inflammation (Toxic Fat Syndrome), the body will preferentially try to store any excess toxic fat (arachidonic acid) in your fat cells (adipose tissue). This is a case of being out of sight and out of harm's way for the rest of the body. That's if you are lucky. If not, the excess toxic fat will continue to circulate throughout the body, spreading increased silent inflammation to every cell in the body. As I discussed in the last chapter, as the levels of AA begin to increase in the adipose tissue, eicosanoids are generated to start making more fat cells to dilute the cellular concentration of incoming AA. You become fatter, but by diluting the levels of AA in any one particular fat cell, you decrease its potential toxicity. At this point, you have a growing adipose tumor, but at least it is benign and not causing any health issues, because the toxic fat is sequestered within the adipose tissue.

The Life of a Fat Cell

If fat cells are healthy, they do their job very effectively. They take up excess calories, store them safely as fat, then release them on command to provide high-octane fuel to make enough adenosine triphosphate (ATP) to keep you alive, with a little extra to allow you to move around. As long as you have healthy fat cells, you are probably not going to have Toxic Fat Syndrome. Depending on your genetics, you might have more trouble getting the high-octane fuel out of the fat cells (the fat trap), but you will have little problem pulling any excess AA out of the bloodstream to prevent inflammatory damage to your other tissues.

The molecular definition of a healthy fat cell is one that can expand and take up excess fat from the blood to prevent lipotoxicity. But genetics determine your release of stored fat. The enzyme (hormone-sensitive lipase) that releases the stored fat is inhibited by insulin. In some people who are genetically lean, this inhibition by insulin is normally low. They will have a hard time accumulating excess body fat because fat is leaving the adipose tissue at virtually the same rate it is entering. These people have a very smoothly running fuel distribution center. These are the genetically lucky ones (or maybe not so lucky, as I will explain later).

Other people have a genetically greater degree of sensitivity to insulin's inhibition of the same enzyme. These are the people who have a fat trap, with fat entering the adipose tissue at a faster rate than it leaves. This is like a warehouse where products are coming in faster than they are going out. The end result is the product piles up inside the warehouse. These people will get fatter even if they are eating the same number of calories as someone who doesn't have a fat trap. It also means they are storing more potential high-octane fuel (fat) in the adipose tissue and can't generate as much ATP for the other cells in the body. Although they have a fat trap, they also have a larger toxic waste dump that may help them live longer.

Sick Fat Cells

Your fat cells start getting sick when they can no longer easily expand to take up any extra fat and especially toxic fat. The primary cause is the increasing levels of AA in the fat cell and the associated silent inflammation that comes with it. Eventually, if the levels of AA become high enough in any one fat cell, then cell death can occur.

Although there is a correlation between excess weight and diabetes, this is not the same as excess weight causing diabetes. If you don't have pre-diabetes (metabolic syndrome) or type 2 diabetes, then the likelihood of premature death due to excess weight is very low. But if you are fat and have Toxic Fat Syndrome, then the correlation between excess weight and mortality becomes very strong.

Below that critical threshold of AA in a fat cell, the response of adipose tissue when exposed to more AA is to make more fat cells to encapsulate incoming AA. Above the critical AA threshold in any particular fat cell, it becomes progressively sicker until it dies. This is the tipping point that turns a benign adipose tumor into a malignant one. Once a fat cell dies, your troubles begin to dramatically multiply.

The first sign indicating that your fat cells are getting sicker is an increase in insulin levels (hyperinsulinemia), which is caused by insulin resistance (explained in detail in appendix F) that starts first in your adipose tissue and then spreads to your muscle cells. With these increased insulin levels comes the appearance of a group of symptoms (such as increased waist circumference, low HDL cholesterol, and high triglycerides) that is called metabolic syndrome, which you could consider pre-diabetes. A 2007 study from Harvard Medical School indicates a strong correlation between the levels of toxic fat in the adipose tissue and the development of metabolic syndrome. As the fat cells become more inflamed, they develop insulin resistance, and the stored toxic fat begins leaking into the bloodstream. Now the muscle cells begin incorporating toxic fat as inflammatory lipid droplets, and insulin resistance starts to develop in those cells. The result is the pancreas starts producing more insulin (hyperinsulinemia) to try to overcome the insulin resistance in the muscle cells. It is hyperinsulinemia that drives the development of metabolic syndrome. Unfortunately, hyperinsulinemia also increases the efficiency of the fat trap in genetically susceptible individuals.

Metabolic syndrome precedes the development of type 2 diabetes by eight to ten years if not reversed. You can't simply look at a person to determine if they have metabolic syndrome, but their blood will tell. If you do have metabolic syndrome or diabetes, you will have a greater chance of mortality at an earlier age. On the other hand, if you have normal insulin, blood glucose, and blood lipid levels, then excess weight will have very little effect on your lifespan as excess toxic fat (AA) remains sequestered in the adipose tissue.

As more fat cells die in the adipose tissue, the development of insulin resistance accelerates throughout the adipose tissue. Stored AA as well as other inflammatory mediators rapidly spill out of the dead fat cells, causing insulin resistance in the nearby cells of the adipose tissue. Insulin's inhibition of the hormone-sensitive lipase is decreased, and now stored fat rich in AA begins streaming into the bloodstream.

This is what I term *malignant toxic fat* because once it enters the bloodstream, it becomes malignant like a cancer and spreads rapidly throughout the body. In cancer, this is known as metastasis. The adipose tissue is ground zero for the metastasic spread of toxic fat. The result is constant inflammatory attacks on all other organs, causing the development of chronic disease at a far earlier age than expected.

Yes, if you have high levels of silent inflammation in the blood, your life is going to be a mess. If you are fat and have excess AA stored in your adipose tissue, you may not be ill, but you are walking on eggshells—this stored AA can become malignant if the levels of AA rise beyond the tipping point in the fat cells to cause their cellular death.

Your real goal in this situation is to first reduce the levels of AA in your adipose tissue, making it more difficult for it to ever become malignant toxic fat. This is especially true if you are considering undertaking a calorie-restricted diet to lose weight. One of the first things that happens with rapid weight loss is the release of stored AA (as well as toxins such as PCBs, dioxins, herbicides, pesticides, and other fat-soluble chemicals) from the fat cells into the bloodstream. The result is a rapid increase in the levels of systemic silent inflammation as you initially lose weight.

If you don't reduce inflammation in the adipose tissue before you start to reduce your calorie intake, you will have an extremely difficult time losing excess fat even if you do "eat less and exercise more" because of increased AA in your bloodstream.

I define the various stages of a silent inflammation-induced adipose tumor much like cancer is described:

Normal: Tumor-free (You are lean, and the blood is not inflamed)

Stage 1: Benign tumor (You are fat, but the blood is not inflamed)

Stage 2: Slowly spreading tumor (You are lean, and the blood is inflamed)

Stage 3: Malignant tumor (You are fat, and the blood is inflamed)

The spread of toxic fat throughout the body resembles the growth of a tumor. It can be encapsulated in the primary tumor (stage 1 tumor), or it can be slow (stage 2 tumor), or a rapidly spreading (stage 3 tumor) cancer. Stage 2 and stage 3 represent different levels of the intensity of Toxic Fat Syndrome.

All cancers start with a primary tumor. As long as the tumor is confined to a specific area and doesn't affect any organ function, it is considered benign. Thus being overweight or even obese with normal blood chemistry (especially relative to the markers of metabolic syndrome) indicates that you have a benign adipose tumor that is growing but may also be acting as a protective mechanism to suck up as much extra AA as possible to prevent its spread to other organs.

Thinking of excess fat as a potentially malignant tumor should scare you as much as any form of cancer. Bottom line: if you are fat and inflamed, the more likely you probably are going to die at an earlier age. Here lies the real linkage between excess fat and chronic disease. Unfortunately, a growing number of Americans, including millions of children, are falling into this latter category.

Cluster Analysis

Public health experts look for outbreaks of disease that may be related to a common cause by cluster analysis. Whether it is an outbreak of infectious disease (such as HIV) or increased occurrence of cancer, cluster analysis is universally applied. In almost every lecture to the general public about obesity, you see a series of slides that show the increasing percentage of obesity in various states. As these slides flash across the screen, it looks a lot like the spread of an infectious disease. But on closer inspection, you see that the spread is led by the states that have the highest levels of poor people.

According to an economic law known as Engle's Law, the less disposable income you have, the more of that income goes to purchase food. The cheapest sources of calories are processed foods rich in refined carbohydrates (which increase insulin) and vegetable oils (which are rich in omega-6 fatty acids). When these two food components are consumed together, they cause increased silent inflammation due to increased AA formation. To protect itself from increased systemic inflammation, the body initially responds by increasing the size of the toxic waste dump (the adipose tissue) in an effort to dilute this growing potential burden of increased silent inflammation. In other words, you get fatter.

You can liken the growth of obesity in America to the growth of Wal-Mart, starting in the poorer rural areas and advancing throughout the country. Whether it is low prices on foods rich in refined carbohydrates and vegetable oils or toys from China, those with the least amount of disposable income are economically driven to maximize the money they have. And when applied to food consumption, it means an increase in silent inflammation.

The Danger of Yo-Yo Weight Changes

Once you begin to lose weight, your fat cells shrink. That's the good news. The bad news is that these shrinking fat cells are releasing stored AA (as well as other stored fat-soluble toxins like PCBs and dioxins) into the bloodstream, forcing your liver to work overtime to try to clear these toxins from the blood. As a result, you aren't going to feel that great during the initial phases of your diet. (Small wonder that most people give up on diets after a few weeks.)

Losing weight and the unavoidable short-term release of stored AA is worth it because of the benefits of completely removing both excess AA and other toxins from your body. But for most people, 95 percent of the initial weight loss is regained at a much faster rate than it was lost. The speed of this weight gain is governed by increasing levels of insulin that come from eating either too many carbohydrates or too many calories (usually a combination of both). Unfortunately, this increased insulin also causes the body to produce more AA. So now with the regained weight, the levels of AA in the stored fat become even greater than before, pushing the adipose tissue to a much higher level of inflammation and therefore greater potential to generate malignant toxic fat.

As you keep yo-yo dieting (losing weight and gaining it back), you are constantly filling your body with increasing levels of AA, which eventually means a constant inflammatory attack on key organs, such as the heart, brain, and immune system. That means more heart disease, Alzheimer's, and cancer. A 2007 European study demonstrated that men who had gone through yo-yo changes in their weight had a much greater likelihood of death compared to those who remained weight stable even if they were obese.

And consider this: the adipose tissue also stores large amounts of other environmental toxins, such as PCBs, dioxins, herbicides, and pesticides that are fat-soluble. When you start losing fat, those toxins are dropped into the bloodstream. If the fat loss is slow (about a pound per week), the liver can convert them into water-soluble compounds that can be excreted from the body. If not, then they go to the next organ that is rich in fat. That's the brain—the last place you want toxins to be stored.

Can Normal-Weight People Have Toxic Fat Syndrome?

The answer is a frightening yes. Being normal weight appears to be a good thing, and it is unless you are producing too much AA. Normally, the buffering capacity of the adipose tissue for fatty acid uptake in those individuals is limited because they have a very efficient distribution that is sending fat out as high-octane fuel as quickly as it comes in. That efficiency becomes a problem if there is an excess amount of AA being produced by the body. Because of the limited capacity of the adipose tissue to absorb it (due to a lack of a fat trap), this becomes a potentially dangerous situation. With no place to store this extra AA, it spreads to other organs, slowly increasing their levels of silent inflammation. This is the underlying process of chronic disease development. This is why it is possible for people who look great in a swimsuit to sometimes have high levels of silent inflammation.

The best example of this type of paradox is that many of the Olympic athletes with whom I have worked over the years have had relatively high levels of silent inflammation due to overtraining, causing increased inflammatory damage throughout their bodies. They looked great physically, but they were far from being well. Once their levels of silent inflammation in the blood were reduced, their performance improved, as did their future prospects for a longer life.

Once you understand that excess fat is an adipose tissue tumor, you realize our obesity epidemic is more complex and potentially a lot more dangerous. Ideally, you want to be at your ideal normal weight *and* not inflamed. This is an indication that you have a very efficient fat redistribution system and are not overproducing toxic fat (AA) from your diet. Unfortunately, few Americans meet these criteria. Most Americans fall into one of three conditions.

Fat and not inflamed. You can view this condition as a temporarily safe holding pattern. But having a benign tumor that is growing more concentrated in AA is dangerous. Consider this situation as stage 1 cancer. Your first task should be the reduction of the excess AA in that benign tumor so that fat cells remain healthy to prevent the rapid spread of stored AA into the bloodstream. This is best done by using the combination of the Zone Diet and high-dose fish oil to reduce the existing inflammation in the adipose tissue.

Normal weight and inflamed. People can also be at their ideal normal weight and inflamed, and that's definitely not good. This can be viewed as a stage 2 tumor with toxic fat slowly spreading to other tissues because it is being produced at a faster rate than the adipose tissue can sequester it, due to a very efficient fat redistribution system. More ominously, no visual clue of Toxic Fat Syndrome is evident. This gives people a real sense of false security, yet this is how most cancers grow. There is often no indication of the presence of the cancer until the diagnosis of an advanced chronic disease.

Fat and inflamed. This is akin to having one foot in the grave and the other foot on a banana peel. Your toxic fat is now spreading rapidly throughout the body. This is a stage 3 adipose tumor and just as dangerous as any other malignant tumor. This situation needs immediate attention, just like any malignant cancer, as time is quickly running out. In stage 3, the dam has basically broken, and the stored AA is rapidly escaping from the adipose tissue, dramatically increasing the intensity of inflammatory attacks on every organ in the body.

The first clinical sign of a stage 3 tumor is the appearance of type 2 diabetes. The 250 percent increase in type 2 diabetes in the past twenty-five years shows that stage 3 adipose tumors are increasing in our country. If any other cancer increased by that level, it would be cause for national outrage but, apparently, not for adipose tumors.

Summary

Understanding that our current obesity crisis is really a cancer epidemic is frightening. Excess AA appears first in the adipose tissue, which acts as a toxic waste dump to prevent excess silent inflammation from circulating in the blood. The containment of this toxic fat can be breached due to insulin resistance in the adipose tissue. This is caused by a progressive sickening of otherwise healthy fat cells as AA accumulates in these cells. When good fat turns bad, the stored toxic fat (AA) is released into the bloodstream, which sets the molecular stage to begin the inflammatory attack on the rest of the organs. Just like a cancer, you feel no pain until enough accumulated damage occurs to begin causing organ failure.

Unlike cancer, however, blood tests that I will describe in the next chapter can tell you years ahead of actual development of chronic disease that Toxic Fat Syndrome is present. The sooner you know, the easier it becomes to reverse the potential damage.

CHAPTER 7

Do You Have Toxic Fat Syndrome?

IT IS VERY DIFFICULT TO TREAT TOXIC FAT SYNDROME IF YOU CAN'T measure it. And until a few years ago, no one could. Because no pain is associated with silent inflammation, few physicians realize it even exists. In fact, the only way you can measure it is from the blood. Olympic athletes can be wracked by silent inflammation, and some overweight people may have very little. Obviously, looks can be deceiving. It's similar to cholesterol testing: only the blood will tell. But if you are like me, you probably greatly dislike having your blood taken for tests.

So are there subjective markers of Toxic Fat Syndrome that might alert you to its presence?

Subjective Markers

Once silent inflammation builds in the bloodstream, you have Toxic Fat Syndrome. Every organ in the body is now under constant inflammatory attack. Over the years, I have developed a number of subjective markers to indicate the potential presence of Toxic Fat Syndrome. As I described earlier, no one marker is sufficient, but if you can answer yes to more than three of these questions, you probably have some degree of Toxic Fat Syndrome. Here is a review of the indicators:

1. Are you overweight?
2. Are you taking a cholesterol-lowering drug?
3. Are you groggy upon waking?
4. Are you prone to stress?
5. Are you constantly craving carbohydrates?
6. Are you fatigued throughout the day?
7. Are you especially hungry two hours after dinner?
8. Are your fingernails brittle?

These seemingly unrelated markers provide a unique insight into your potential for having Toxic Fat Syndrome. So let's examine each independently.

Overweight

The first question is how to define your ideal weight. The use of measurements such as BMI is often misleading, because many elite athletes (especially those in sports requiring strength) have a BMI that would rank them as overweight. This is because a pound of muscle occupies less space than a pound of fat. Likewise many people with apparently normal BMIs have high levels of Toxic Fat Syndrome.

One good measure of what your ideal weight should be is what it was at age twenty. By that time, your growth has stopped, and you have maximum levels of testosterone that build muscle mass. Your body composition will change as you age (so the clothes you wore at age twenty will not fit as well as you age), even if you weigh exactly the same.

Here is another marker of your ideal weight: your waist size (measured at the belly button) should be about half your height. You can almost hear a collective groan from most Americans for both of my definitions of ideal body weight.

However, the most objective measurement of your ideal weight is your percent body fat. The most efficient calculation method of doing this at home uses a tape measure, a scale, and few tables. The tables can be found in the body fat calculator on my Web site at www.drsears.com (under Zone Resources), but in general, the ideal percentage of body fat for a male should be about 15 percent. At this level, you will not have any love handles. For a female, the ideal percentage of body fat should be about 22 percent. At this percentage of body fat, you should not have any cellulite. Models whose abdominal muscles are prominent have body fat measuring less than 10 percent for males and less than 15 percent for females. This is simply an unrealistic goal for most normal individuals and not necessary for good health. And once the body fat levels dip below 6 percent for males and below 13 percent for females, it becomes an unhealthy situation.

If you are overweight by any of these definitions, then you definitely have silent inflammation. However, it may not have spread beyond your adipose tissue into the bloodstream. If it hasn't, then you have a benign adipose tumor and no sign of Toxic Fat Syndrome—yet.

Taking Cholesterol-Lowering Drugs

Statins are the only drugs known to increase arachidonic acid (AA) formation and hence increase Toxic Fat Syndrome. This may explain why one of the main side effects of these drugs is short-term memory loss, due to inflammation in the brain as well as lowering cholesterol levels in the nerves needed to maintain neural transmission.

Groggy upon Waking

Re-establishing the correct neurotransmitter balance is one of the reasons you need to sleep. Increased levels of the eicosanoids derived from AA in the brain can interfere with that process.

Prone to Stress

Stress is simply any change to your physiological or emotional environment. The degree of your response to stress is dependent on your levels of AA-derived eicosanoids. The higher their levels, the more sensitive you are to various stressors.

Constantly Craving Carbohydrates

This is an indication of insulin resistance and abnormally high blood insulin levels. The elevated insulin drives down blood glucose levels rapidly, forcing the brain into a panic situation where it tells you to eat more carbohydrates as soon as possible. Excess insulin also drives the formation of AA, especially if you are consuming a diet rich in carbohydrates and vegetable oils but low in fish oil (that is, the Perfect Nutritional Storm).

Constant Fatigue

This can be a combination of both mental and physical fatigue. The mental fatigue is caused by excess levels of AA in the brain. The physical fatigue is caused by the lack of sufficient adenosine triphosphate (ATP) formation for muscle and metabolic needs because insulin is preventing the release of high-octane fuel (fat) from your fat cells to be used as an energy source to make ATP.

Exceptionally Hungry Two Hours after Dinner

Hunger a few hours after eating dinner is an indicator of increased endocannabinoid levels in the brain activating their receptors and creating the munchies.

Brittle Fingernails, Limp Hair

Pro-inflammatory eicosanoids inhibit the production of the structural protein keratin in the fingernails and hair. Without enough keratin, your nails become brittle and hair limp.

If you answered positively to more than three of these questions, it is worth your while to begin to consider looking at the true markers of silent inflammation that can only be found in the blood.

Blood Markers for Toxic Fat Syndrome

Most people hate to give blood. That's why they have their annual physical check-up every five years—if not longer. However, whenever you do have your physical, the doctor usually does a fasting lipid test. This could offer the first clue that you may have Toxic Fat Syndrome. Focus on two of the numbers on that test: the level of triglycerides (TG) and the level of HDL (good) cholesterol.

Now divide the level of triglycerides by the HDL cholesterol to get a ratio. If the TG/HDL ratio is greater than 4, then you probably have

Toxic Fat Syndrome. The TG/HDL ratio is a marker for insulin resistance and the cluster of conditions known as metabolic syndrome. The higher the TG/HDL ratio, the greater the degree of insulin resistance you have. If you have insulin resistance, the encapsulated AA in your adipose tissue is already leaking into your bloodstream and beginning its relentless inflammatory attack on your other organs.

If you have a high TG/HDL ratio, it's time to consider another blood test for your fasting insulin level. If your fasting insulin level is high (greater than 10 uU/ml), you are increasing the activity of the enzyme (delta-5-desaturase) that is key in the production of AA. A good number for fasting insulin is under 10 uU/ml; less than 5 uU/ml is ideal. The lower your fasting insulin levels, the longer and better you are going to live. Lowering insulin is one of the primary benefits of the Zone Diet.

However, you can have a low TG/HDL ratio and low insulin and still have Toxic Fat Syndrome. This is often the case with elite athletes or anyone who does a lot of exercise.

The final confirmatory test for Toxic Fat Syndrome comes from the fatty acid composition of the blood, and in particular the levels of the essential fatty acid precursors of eicosanoids.

As I mentioned earlier, only three fatty acids can be transformed into eicosanoids, the hormones that control inflammation: arachidonic acid (AA), dihomo-gamma-linolenic acid (DGLA), and eicosapentaenoic acid (EPA). From AA come all the pro-inflammatory eicosanoids that in excess accelerate chronic disease. From DGLA come very powerful anti-inflammatory eicosanoids that accelerate cellular rejuvenation. Finally, from EPA come neutral eicosanoids, but the presence of EPA can partially inhibit the synthesis of AA as well as dilute AA concentration in the cell membrane, making it more difficult to make pro-inflammatory eicosanoids. The balance of these three fatty acids in the blood will tell your future with laser-like precision. If you take only one blood test in your life, this should be the test as it provides the earliest clinical sign that you can no longer be considered well. Initially, what you are looking for are the following fatty acid levels:

- ➤ AA less than 9 percent of total fatty acids
- ➤ DGLA greater than 3 percent of total fatty acids
- ➤ EPA greater than 4 percent of total fatty acids

These absolute numbers of the individual fatty acids are only your first indicator that you may have Toxic Fat Syndrome. However, it is the ratio of these fatty acids to each other that tells the full story. The true marker of Toxic Fat Syndrome is the AA/EPA ratio. If it is greater than 10, then you have Toxic Fat Syndrome, regardless of how good you look in a swimsuit. A good ratio is 3, and the ideal ratio is about 1.5.

Where did I get these numbers? The people who live the longest today are the Japanese. They also have the longest health span (longevity minus years of disability) as well as the lowest levels of heart disease in industrialized countries. Finally, you shouldn't be too surprised to learn that the Japanese have the lowest rates of depression in the world. When you look at the blood of the Japanese population, the AA/EPA ratio ranges from 1.5 to 3. (Note that these are Japanese people living in Japan, not people of Japanese heritage who are living in other countries.) The average "healthy" American has an AA/EPA ratio greater than 12, whereas Europeans in the Mediterranean region have ratios between 6 and 9. This means Americans are not only the fattest people in the world today but also the most inflamed. If you have chronic disease, it is likely that your AA/EPA ratio is greater than 20.

This fatty acid test is not a standard test, however. Although it is often used in research applications, most physicians are still totally unaware of it. In appendix B, I list some laboratories that do such testing.

> Can your arachidonic acid (AA)/eicosapentaenoic acid (EPA) ratio be too low? Yes. If the AA/EPA ratio is too low, you may not be able to mount an appropriate inflammatory response when you need to. If the ratio is about 0.7 (as it is in the native Eskimo population), you will be more prone to infections. If it drops to 0.5, the risk of hemorrhagic stroke increases. This is why I like to keep the lower limit of the AA/EPA ratio to 1.5, as found in the native Japanese population.
>
> The AA/EPA ratio is a measure of the pro-inflammatory potential of your cells. The higher the AA/EPA ratio, the greater the amount of silent inflammation you have in your organs, which indicates you are moving quickly toward the development of some type of chronic disease associated with Toxic Fat Syndrome. The result is that you will age faster and lose your wellness more rapidly.

What About C-Reactive Protein?

We hear a lot these days about a protein known as C-reactive protein (CRP) as a marker of inflammation. Unfortunately, it is a very non-specific marker of silent inflammation that can rise rapidly with acute infections. In fact, a study published in the 2004 issue of the *New England Journal of Medicine* indicated that CRP levels don't provide any more real significant predictive value in the treatment of heart disease than traditional risk factors. Elevated blood levels of the AA/EPA ratio (the marker of Toxic Fat Syndrome) can show up years before constantly elevated levels of CRP are observed. By the time CRP becomes constantly elevated, you have had Toxic Fat Syndrome for a long time. Consider the AA/EPA ratio as your early warning system that you are suffering from Toxic Fat Syndrome and can no longer be considered well.

Markers of Malignant Toxic Fat	
Test	
AA/EPA ratio	greater than 15
Fasting Insulin (uU/ml)	greater than 15
TG/HDL ratio	greater than 4

Notice that body weight is not one of the markers. This is because you can be normal weight yet have a high AA/EPA ratio, which indicates the slow spread of toxic fat. You wouldn't be considered fat, but you are definitely not well, although the toxic fat has not yet become malignant (a stage 3 tumor). But if you have the markers of malignant toxic fat, you have to take immediate dietary steps (the combination of the Zone Diet (see chapter 8) and high-dose fish oil (see chapter 9) to reverse it, since there is no drug that can lower it.

If you are overweight and all your clinical markers are in the low-risk range, this doesn't let you off the hook because the encapsulated AA stored in your fat cells can become malignant at any time. This is the ideal time to start working on reducing the size of your benign adipose tumor using the anti-inflammatory Zone dietary program.

Measuring Your Anti-Aging Potential

Keeping silent inflammation under control is only half of your life-long wellness strategy. You also have to have a reserve of anti-inflammatory potential to maximize the rejuvenation of your cells. Consider this anti-inflammatory potential as your anti-aging reservoir.

Nothing makes physicians cringe more than hearing the term "anti-aging" medicine. Because aging is natural, the term is an oxymoron. However, if you replace the phrase "anti-aging" with "anti-inflammatory," then even Harvard Medical School welcomes you with open arms. Yet the goal of both disciplines is the same: to increase the body's ability to rejuvenate itself at a faster rate.

These cellular rejuvenation mechanisms are deeply imbedded in your genes, and decreasing the AA/DGLA ratio in every cell in the body can activate them. This ensures that you are increasing the likelihood of making more good eicosanoids (from DGLA) and fewer bad ones (from AA). The better you do that, the more effectively your cells can rejuvenate themselves.

The lower the AA/DGLA ratio, the greater the potential to make good eicosanoids to enhance wellness and essentially reverse aging. (You can find the scientific basis for that cellular rejuvenation in one of my earlier books, *The Anti-Aging Zone*.)

Markers of Wellness

The good news is that the clinical markers that describe the extent of Toxic Fat Syndrome can also become clinical markers that quantify wellness. Standard blood tests show how sick we are, but what you really want are blood tests that tell how well you are. Here are the two most important numbers you should know:

AA/EPA ratio less than 3 (but no less than 1.5)

AA/DGLA ratio less than 3

The AA/EPA ratio is the best marker of Toxic Fat Syndrome and can be summarized in the following table:

Dangerously High	Poor	Good	Ideal	Too Low
Greater than 15	10	3	1.5	Less than 0.75

If the AA/EPA is higher than 15, then you are rapidly accelerating yourself toward the early development of chronic disease. At 1.5, you have an ideal balance. Below 0.75, you may not have enough inflammatory reserve to effectively fight infections. In essence, there is a zone of inflammation that you want to maintain.

Likewise your cellular rejuvenation potential is best determined by the AA/DGLA ratio. Ideally, it should be less than 3. The higher the AA/DGLA ratio, the less ability you have to reverse the effects of aging.

Wellness can be defined as finding the right balance of both your body's ability to control inflammation caused by external causes (infections, injury, and diet) as well as its ability to generate internal anti-inflammatory responses necessary for cellular rejuvenation. Ideally, this would be monitored by simply measuring eicosanoid levels in the blood. Unfortunately, eicosanoids don't circulate in the blood because they are cell-to-cell regulators. However, their precursors (DGLA, AA, and EPA) do circulate in the blood and can be measured. It is the balance of these essential fatty acids to each other that gives you a powerful insight into your current state of wellness.

Other Markers of Wellness

While the ratios of these three fatty acids (DGLA, AA, and EPA) determine the status of inflammation potential (both pro- and anti-inflammation) in your body, they are not the only markers of wellness. Another important one is your degree of insulin resistance. As I explain in appendix F, insulin resistance not only increases AA production by increasing insulin levels but also accelerates the release of toxic fat stored in your adipose tissue to the rest of your organs via the bloodstream. The best marker for insulin resistance is your fasting insulin level.

Unfortunately, most physicians rarely measure fasting insulin levels. But you can find one last marker of wellness in every standard blood test: the ratio of fasting triglycerides to HDL cholesterol. Consider the TG/HDL ratio as the poor man's marker of insulin resistance.

So here is your complete wellness scorecard:

	Dangerous	Poor	Good	Ideal
Silent Inflammation Status				
AA/EPA ratio	> 15	10	3	1.5
Insulin Resistance Status				
Fasting insulin	> 15 uU/ml	10 uU/ml	5 uU/ml	<5 uU/ml
TG/HDL ratio	> 4	3	2	< 1

This is not a multiple-choice test. Either you pass all the tests, or you can't be considered well. And here is why looks can be deceiving. As I said earlier, virtually every Olympic athlete with whom I have worked had high levels of silent inflammation because they train too hard. They look great in swimsuits, but they aren't well. Once they lower their levels of silent inflammation, they perform at a much higher level. This may help to explain why the athletes with whom I have personally worked have won twenty-four gold medals in the past four Olympics. They had a powerful hormonal advantage.

Summary

The appearance of Toxic Fat Syndrome in the bloodstream is the indication that silent inflammation is beginning to attack your organs. You can't feel it, but you can measure it. As your levels of Toxic Fat Syndrome increase, a complex series of biological events are set in motion, giving rise to increased inflammatory attack on every organ throughout your body. The result is the accelerated development of chronic disease. There is no drug that can reverse silent inflammation, but there are dietary tools that enable you to begin to reverse Toxic Fat Syndrome in less than thirty days. What these tools are and how they can be used are described in the following chapters.

CHAPTER 8

The Zone Diet: Your Primary Defense in Fighting Toxic Fat

THE KEY FACTOR THAT CONTRIBUTES TO TOXIC FAT SYNDROME is the body's levels of excess arachidonic acid (AA). In high enough concentrations, this natural fatty acid is exceptionally toxic. Yet the only thing that governs the amount of AA in your body is your diet. I developed the Zone Diet more than twenty years ago for one purpose—to reduce the levels of toxic fat and by doing so reduce the levels of silent inflammation throughout the body.

It's been more than a decade since my first book, *The Zone*, was published, yet sometimes it seems as if no one ever really read the book. To this day, the Zone Diet is still thought of as a weight-loss program. It is a diet, in the truest sense of the word. The root word for *diet* comes from the ancient Greek meaning "way of life." The Zone Diet is simply a way of life to keep the levels of toxic fat (AA) under control for a lifetime. If we can achieve that goal, then we have essentially eliminated Toxic Fat Syndrome. At the same time, people will lose weight because it is silent inflammation in both the adipose tissue and in the brain that drives our epidemic of obesity.

The Role of Hormones in Weight Loss

Losing weight is incredibly easy as long as you are never hungry. Scientifically, lack of hunger is called satiety, and ultimately your hormones control it. If you can keep these hormones that are directly affected by what you eat within a zone that is not too high but not too low, then you are guaranteed the following:

- ➤ You will not be hungry between meals.
- ➤ You will have peak mental and physical performance throughout the day.
- ➤ You will lose excess body fat at the fastest possible rate.
- ➤ You will decrease silent inflammation.
- ➤ You will reverse Toxic Fat Syndrome.

The first two benefits of the Zone Diet are relatively immediate benefits that are easily observed within a matter of days. The loss of excess body fat will take longer as it is virtually impossible to lose more than 1 to 1.5 pounds of excess fat per week (although your clothes will be fitting better). The last two benefits represent your pathway back to wellness and can only be determined by the blood tests described in the previous chapter.

Hunger and Satiety

Hunger is probably the most powerful urge we have. When you are truly hungry, everything else (including sex) becomes secondary because the brain is desperate for the energy it needs to function. On the other hand, satiety can be just as powerful. The brain's energy needs are being met, and you now have more important things to do than constantly search for food.

Our current obesity epidemic is a result of these two opposing powerful forces (hunger and satiety) being out of balance. Hormones control that balance of hunger and satiety, especially the ones directly affected by the diet, and in particular by the Zone Diet.

Insulin, Obesity, and Inflammation

As I said earlier, it is excess insulin that makes you fat and keeps you fat. How insulin does that is a little more complex.

There are two ways to increase insulin levels in your body: eating too many carbohydrates and eating too many calories. Americans have been doing both for the past twenty-five years. However, not everyone who eats too many calories or carbohydrates has become fat.

Virtually all cells in the body have receptors for insulin. Insulin resistance occurs when the binding of insulin to these receptors doesn't result in the correct signal being transmitted to a particular cell. If the insulin resistance occurs in the muscle cell, then your muscles can't effectively take up glucose from the bloodstream. Because excess glucose in the blood is toxic, the body responds by secreting even more insulin, and finally enough insulin is available in the blood to drive down blood glucose levels by brute force. Unfortunately, the same high levels of insulin now drive the liver to make more AA, especially if your diet is rich in omega-6 fatty acids. Now you have even more toxic fat (AA) floating in the bloodstream that needs to be removed. If it is not rapidly removed, then you will have the beginning of Toxic Fat Syndrome.

Just to illustrate how toxic AA can be: You can inject excess levels of virtually any fatty acid into a rabbit and nothing adverse will happen. You can even inject excess cholesterol, and the rabbit will be okay. But if you inject excess AA into the same rabbit, the animal will be dead within minutes.

Excess insulin makes it easier to produce AA from excess dietary omega-6 fatty acids. Unless you can take this excess AA out of the bloodstream and deposit it in your adipose tissue, that AA will continue to circulate until another organ takes it up, causing inflammatory damage at the molecular level.

Glycemic Index and Glycemic Load

To understand how both protein and carbohydrates work together to control hunger and satiety, and in the process control silent inflammation, you have to start with understanding the relationship of the glycemic index and the glycemic load to excess insulin formation.

In the old days, nutritional advice was a lot easier with respect to carbohydrates. Complex carbohydrates (such as potatoes and bread) were good because they were thought to slowly enter the bloodstream, whereas simple carbohydrates (such as table sugar) were "bad" because they were thought to enter the bloodstream more rapidly. It was so obvious that there was no need to clinically confirm such an obvious truth. That was until someone actually did the human experiments. That person was David Jenkins in the early 1980s, and the world of nutrition was suddenly turned upside down. Some complex carbohydrates (such as potatoes) were entering the bloodstream as glucose at a much faster rate than simple carbohydrates (such as table sugar). For the past twenty-five years, this concept has been hotly debated primarily by those who have built their reputations on the premise that complex carbohydrates are good and simple ones are bad, no matter what the facts are.

The real key to understanding how carbohydrates affect insulin is not measured by the glycemic index of a carbohydrate (that is, how fast a defined amount (50 g) of carbohydrate enters the bloodstream as glucose) but by the glycemic load in a meal. To figure glycemic load, you multiply the amount of carbohydrate consumed in the meal by that carbohydrate's glycemic index (which you can find on the Internet). Now you have a far better indicator of how much insulin will be secreted in response to that meal. As shown by researchers at Harvard Medical School in the late 1990s, the higher the glycemic load, the more likely you are to become fat, become diabetic, develop heart disease, and be inflamed.

What is the best way to reduce the glycemic load of the diet? Eat a lot of colorful nonstarchy vegetables, such as green beans, broccoli, and spinach; consume a limited amount of fruits, such as berries or apples; and significantly cut back on the consumption of grains and starches. These are the basic recommendations of the Zone Diet that I made in 1995. Making those seemingly simple changes will reduce the glycemic load of the diet and, as a result, decrease insulin secretion and reduce the resulting production of toxic fat.

Protein and Satiety

The Zone Diet is more complex than simply reducing the glycemic load of the diet. You also have to balance the reduced glycemic load with the appropriate amount of protein at each meal. You need protein to induce satiety. The first role of protein is to stimulate the hormone glucagon that stabilizes blood glucose levels, thus reducing hunger. The second role of protein is to stimulate the release of a hormone known as PYY (peptide YY) from the gut that goes directly to the brain to tell you to stop eating. If you aren't hungry, then cutting back on calories is easy.

So exactly how much protein do you need at each meal to create satiety? It would be the size and thickness of the palm of your hand. That's about 3 ounces of low-fat protein for a typical female and about 4 ounces of low-fat protein for a typical male. Of course, you need to control the glycemic load of the meal at the same time.

Fat and Inflammation

The other key factor for the success of the Zone Diet as an anti-inflammatory diet is the vigorous restriction of the omega-6 fatty acids that have become ubiquitous in our diet. Without a dietary overload of omega-6 fatty acids, it becomes very difficult to make excess AA even with elevated insulin levels. In essence, by reducing the intake of omega-6 fatty acids, you are choking off the production of AA regardless of the amount of insulin you have in the bloodstream. This is why the primary fats recommended for the Zone Diet are those rich in monounsaturated fats. Products such as olive oil, slivered almonds, and guacamole are typical choices rich in monounsaturated fats. Frankly, they taste a lot better than corn, soybean, safflower, and sunflower oils (all rich in omega-6 fatty acids), and their use radically reduces the dietary supply of the omega-6 fatty acid building blocks required to make AA. Once you reduce AA levels throughout the body, Toxic Fat Syndrome begins to recede.

Unlike protein, dietary fat doesn't have nearly the impact on satiety hormones as glucagon and PYY. But by making monounsaturated fat the primary fat source in the diet, you can indirectly affect a group of brain hormones that promote hunger. These are the endocannabinoids, which are derived from AA. As AA levels are reduced throughout the body (including the brain), endocannabinoids in the brain are also reduced. As you reduce the levels of endocannabinoids, you also reduce hunger.

Thus the seemingly simple dietary recommendations of the Zone Diet contain some very subtle hormonal responses as listed below:

> Lowering the glycemic load of each meal reduces insulin secretion, which helps maintain stable blood glucose levels as well as reduce the activation of the enzyme (delta-5-desaturase) that produces toxic fat.

> Protein stimulates the hormone glucagon from the pancreas. Glucagon in turn stimulates the liver to release stored carbohydrate to help maintain blood sugar levels. As a result, blood sugar levels are further stabilized and the brain is happy. Glucagon also inhibits the activity of the enzyme that makes AA. Protein also stimulates another hormone (PYY) from the gut that goes directly to the brain and generates satiety signals in the hypothalamus.

> The replacement of omega-6 fats with monounsaturated fats chokes off the levels of incoming dietary building blocks required for the formation of AA.

The end result of making Zone meals is that you are not hungry for the next four to six hours because you have balanced the glycemic load of a meal with the appropriate amount of low-fat protein.

The Zone Diet Made Real Easy

Preparing Zone meals is a lot easier than you think. I have developed a number of systems over the years that vary according to how much time and effort you want to expend.

Listed below are my various food accounting systems:

➤ Think Method
➤ Hand-Eye Method
➤ 1-2-3 Method
➤ Food Block Method

The Think Method

Just thinking about balancing protein with carbohydrate is a major step. In other words, never consume carbohydrate without a protein chaser. You may not make the correct balance, but at least you are thinking about it. Say you have a compelling urge to eat a candy bar. If you decide to eat it, have some protein, such as a piece of cheese, to balance it. (Actually, it will take about four ounces of cheese to balance out the candy bar, but more on that later.) If you have an alcoholic drink, always have a protein chaser. A glass of wine and a piece of cheese or a bottle of beer and four chicken wings are good examples.

How do you know if you were successful? Simply look at your watch. If you aren't hungry four hours later, then your thinking has paid off.

The lack of hunger (satiety) is the best indication that what you are eating matches your genetics.

The Hand-Eye Method

This method only requires one hand and one eye to get a lot of hormonal precision. At each meal, simply divide your plate into three equal sections. On one-third of the plate, put enough low-fat protein (chicken, fish, very lean beef, low-fat dairy products, tofu, or soy imitation meat products) to match the size and thickness of your palm. Obviously the larger your hand, the more low-fat protein you get to eat. Realistically, this is about 3 ounces for the typical female, and 4 ounces for the typical male. Now fill the other two-thirds of the plate with low glycemic-load carbohydrates, such as colorful nonstarchy vegetables and fruits (a comprehensive listing can be found in appendix H). What about grains and starches? You use them as condiments (that means small amounts). In general, the more color you see on the plate, the lower the glycemic load of the meal. Finally, add a dash (that's a small amount) of heart-healthy monounsaturated fat, such as olive oil, slivered almonds, or guacamole.

In many ways, the Zone Diet can be viewed as the evolution of the Mediterranean diet. Both diets are rich in vegetables and fruits. Both diets contain adequate, but not excessive, consumption of low-fat protein, such as fish or chicken. Both diets strongly recommend using monounsaturated fats (such as olive oil) as the primary added fat to the diet. Up to this point the Zone Diet and the Mediterranean diet seem identical. There's one very small—but important—exception. On the Zone Diet you significantly cut back (but don't have to totally avoid) grains and starches, and make up for it by eating even more nonstarchy

Mediterranean vegetables and fruits (such as berries). This one seemingly small dietary change has dramatic hormonal consequences. You are reducing the glycemic load of the diet, and in the process you are also reducing insulin levels. This is why the Zone Diet can be considered to be the evolution of a good diet (i.e., the Mediterranean diet) into a hormonally superior diet (i.e., the Zone Diet).

Typical Mediterranean Vegetables	
Nonstarchy (use primarily)	Starchy (use very sparingly)
Artichokes	Corn
Bell peppers	Peas
Broccoli	Potatoes
Eggplant	
Green beans	
Kale	
Onions	
Mushrooms	
Spinach	
Zucchini	
You can see you have a lot of great choices using nonstarchy Mediterranean vegetables.	

The 1-2-3 Method

This method is ideally suited for processed foods that have the nutrition labels on the back of the package. For every *one* gram of fat you eat, you want *two* grams of protein, and *three* grams of carbohydrates. At a meal, the typical female would need about 10 grams of fat, 20 grams of protein, and 30 grams of total carbohydrates (including the fiber). The typical male would need about 15 grams of fat, 30 grams of protein, and 45 grams of carbohydrate per meal (again including fiber, which accounts for about 10 percent of the total carbohydrate). In both cases, they fulfill the 1-2-3 rule.

Once you start looking at the nutrition labels of your favorite processed foods (try starting with pasta or bread), you will quickly see that virtually nothing in the supermarket aisles is remotely close to this Zone balance. Without having that 1-2-3 balance, it is virtually impossible to keep your hormones in the Zone to maintain satiety, which means you will be constantly hungry. Good for the processed food industry, not great for your personal wellness.

The 1-2-3 method is not as precise as the Food Block Method, which is described next, but it's simpler to remember when you're in that supermarket aisle.

The Food Block Method

This is the most accurate method, which subtracts the amount of fiber from the total carbohydrate, as fiber has no effect on insulin secretion. Simply use the hand-eye method to estimate the amount of low-fat protein you need, or follow the Food Block Guide (see appendix H), and then add a dash of heart-healthy monounsaturated fat.

Now your only decision is how much carbohydrate to add. What the Food Block system does is automatically reduce the glycemic load of a meal without you even thinking about it.

The average female will need three Zone Carbohydrate Blocks for a typical meal; the average male needs four per meal. The more low glycemic-load carbohydrates, such as nonstarchy vegetables, you put on your plate, the more food you can eat. But if you choose high glycemic-load carbohydrates, such as grains, bread, and pasta, you will have a lot of empty space on your plate if you want to maintain the correct protein-to-glycemic-load balance needed to control insulin.

Hint: low glycemic-load carbohydrates are also generally the most colorful while most high glycemic-load carbohydrates are without much color and are often white. And if you don't generally like vegetables, then try to focus on vegetables used in Italian cooking. No one ever complains about eating vegetables when visiting Tuscany.

Low Glycemic-Load Carbohydrates	High Glycemic-Load Carbohydrates
Nonstarchy vegetables (broccoli, green beans, peppers, and so forth)	Grains and starches (bread, rice, pasta, and so forth)
Temperate fruits (berries, apples, pears, and so forth)	Tropical fruits (melons, pineapple, and so forth)

Unlike protein and fat, where most people often use only one item at a meal, you can add a variety of Zone Carbohydrate Blocks at each meal. Always try to choose a wide variety of the most colorful carbohydrates.

Appendix H contains a detailed list of both favorable and unfavorable Zone Carbohydrate Blocks as well as Protein and Fat Blocks. This illustrates the flexibility of the Zone Diet, as you never restrict anything from your plate. But treat high glycemic-load carbohydrates like condiments.

You will also refer to the Food Block Guide when you're using the recipes presented in the 28-day meal plans later in this book. Because you can substitute one block for another, you can see the wide variety of meals that can be enjoyed on the Zone Diet. Don't want half an apple? Substitute one peach or half an orange or one-half cup of grapes and so on. Don't like green beans? Instead of one and one-half cups of green beans, have two cups of zucchini or one-quarter cup of kidney beans or two tomatoes and so on. You get the idea.

Zone Rules on Meal Timing

Regardless of what system you use, it's even easier if you follow a few simple rules on meal timing:

1. Eat when you wake up. Always eat within one hour of waking. You have just come off an eight- to ten-hour fast, and your body is on empty.

2. Eat at least every five hours. Don't let more than five hours go by without eating a Zone meal or Zone snack.

3. Eat three meals, two snacks. Have three Zone meals and two Zone snacks in a day. Have a Zone snack between lunch and dinner (that's usually more than five hours for most people) and your final Zone snack before you go to bed, because you won't be eating for the next eight hours.

Does It Work?

In 2000, Harvard Medical School researchers compared the health of men and women who followed the then-current USDA Food Pyramid compared to those who followed diets with higher levels of fruits and vegetables and chicken and fish (a Zone-like diet). They found those who followed the USDA Food Pyramid had higher incidences of heart disease and chronic disease. It's as if the old USDA Food Pyramid was designed to cause a loss of wellness in America by increasing Toxic Fat Syndrome. The new USDA Food Pyramid issued in 2005 is so complex and ill-defined that no one (even at Harvard Medical School) seems to know what it promotes.

Clinical Validation of the Zone Diet

Three things in life are visceral because they are based on belief systems: religion, politics, and nutrition. The true believers of each never want to face any facts that seem to contradict their beliefs, because they know in their hearts they are right. Unlike religion and politics, only nutrition has the potential to be examined scientifically. But you have to ask the right questions and use the right tools. The right question should be:

"What is the best diet to reduce silent inflammation?"

A proper way to study that question would be to give people prepared meals with an equal number of calories with different ratios of protein, carbohydrate, and fat. Essentially you are treating your dietary subjects like lab rats, so they should not be allowed to think about what they are eating. Unfortunately, such clinical trials are very expensive, and as a consequence very few have been published. But the ones that have been published have made one thing very clear: in every study in which diet has been highly controlled, the Zone Diet has been proven to be superior for insulin control, blood sugar control, blood lipid control, appetite suppression, fat loss and, finally, the most important parameter—reduction of silent inflammation.

Reduction of silent inflammation is the most important. In 2004, Harvard Medical School found that the Zone Diet was *nine times* more effective in reducing silent inflammation than the universally recommended USDA Food Pyramid. In addition, I published a study in 2006 that demonstrated that the Atkins diet *doubled* the level of Toxic Fat Syndrome in only six weeks when compared to the Zone Diet, which lowered it. If there were ever a reason *not* to follow the Atkins diet, then increasing Toxic Fat Syndrome would be the primary reason.

Listed below are some of the carefully controlled diet studies that validate the other benefits of the Zone Diet.

Parameter	Study
Insulin control	Dumesnil et al (2001), Layman et al (2003), Pereira et al (2004)
Blood lipid control	Wolfe et al (1999), Dumesnil et al (2001), Layman et al (2003), Fontani et al (2005), Johnston et al (2006)
Blood sugar control	Layman et al (2003), Nuttall et al (2003), Gannon et al (2003)
Fat loss	Skov et al (1999), Layman et al (2003), Fontani et al (2005), Ebbeling et al (2007)
Appetite control	Ludwig et al (1999), Agus et al (2000)
Inflammation control	Pereira et al (2004), Johnson et al (2006)

But the real validation of the Zone Diet occurred in 2005, when the Joslin Diabetes Research Center at Harvard Medical School announced its newest dietary guidelines for treating obesity, pre-diabetes, and type 2 diabetes. What were the new dietary recommendations? Basically those of the Zone Diet.

Who Is Ideally Suited for the Zone Diet?

Obviously, not everyone is genetically identical, so many people believe the Zone Diet can't be the optimal dietary program for everyone. Is that true? Using published research, it is easy to determine who would benefit the most from following the Zone Diet.

Those with existing inflammatory diseases. Because the Zone Diet has been shown to be an anti-inflammatory diet by Harvard Medical School, then it should be the first choice for anyone with an existing chronic disease who has an inflammatory component. That would include cardiovascular patients, cancer patients, Alzheimer's patients, and a long list of others.

Those wishing to reduce silent inflammation. As I mentioned earlier, in carefully controlled studies, the Zone Diet has been shown to be *nine times* more effective than the USDA Food Pyramid in reducing silent inflammation. Likewise the Atkins diet has been shown to double silent inflammation in as little as six weeks compared to the Zone Diet. So if you are interested in reducing silent inflammation, then the Zone Diet is your best choice.

Those with diabetes or glucose intolerance. Since the Zone Diet has been shown to be effective in long-term blood glucose control, anyone with diabetes or glucose intolerance should also benefit from it.

Athletes and active people of normal weight. Because active, normal-weight individuals do better on the Zone Diet than the standard diet recommended to athletes, anyone who is actively exercising and not seeking to lose weight should be on the Zone Diet.

Overweight and obese individuals with a high initial insulin response. Harvard Medical School has shown that overweight or obese people with a high initial insulin secretion response to food (those who release a lot of insulin immediately after eating) will lose far more weight on the Zone Diet than on a low-fat, high-carbohydrate diet with an equal number of calories. This is important since most overweight and obese individuals are insulin resistant and, therefore, have to secrete more insulin after a meal to reduce their blood sugar levels.

Looking at the published data, I would say, if you don't have a chronic disease, aren't concerned about reducing silent inflammation, don't have blood glucose problems, are not actively exercising, and don't have a high initial insulin secretion response to food, then any other diet will probably work in weight loss as well as the Zone Diet. But why take a chance?

Summary

The primary tool for reversing Toxic Fat Syndrome is the Zone Diet because you are *reducing the levels of AA in every cell in the body* by reducing the levels of insulin and restricting the intake of omega-6 fatty acids. In the process, you will lose weight because you will be increasing satiety and decreasing hunger. If you aren't hungry, then cutting back on calories is easy. But if using your hand and your eye to balance your plate at every meal seems too difficult, despite the great health benefits, you still have one last opportunity to reverse Toxic Fat Syndrome, which I describe in the next chapter.

CHAPTER 9

Super Fish Oil: Your Final Defense in Fighting Toxic Fat

I F A TRUE DEFINITION OF A MAGIC BULLET FOR REVERSING TOXIC FAT Syndrome existed, it would have the following qualities:

- ➤ Reduces the consequences of Toxic Fat Syndrome within thirty days
- ➤ Can be taken for a lifetime
- ➤ Has no side effects other than making you smarter
- ➤ Increases cellular rejuvenation at any age

Now this is something that drug companies would love to sell! The only problem is the magic bullet isn't a drug, it doesn't require a prescription, and it has taken me twenty-five years to develop it. This remarkable "wonder drug" is super fish oil (ultra-refined EPA/DHA concentrates that have been enriched with toasted sesame oil concentrate, plus a touch of gamma-linolenic acid, known as GLA). Unlike the Zone Diet, which requires some degree of awareness every time you eat, supplementing your diet with enough super fish oil to help reduce Toxic Fat Syndrome takes only fifteen seconds a day. Both fish oil and super fish oil will reduce Toxic Fat Syndrome to some extent. However, regular fish oil will also reduce your cellular rejuvenation potential, whereas super fish oil will increase it.

All fish oils contain the omega-3 fatty acid, eicosapentaenoic acid (EPA). So if you have trouble reducing arachidonic acid (AA) levels if you aren't strictly following the Zone Diet, you can at least dilute the excess AA being induced by the Perfect Nutritional Storm by increasing the levels of EPA in every cell in the body. This essentially decreases the likelihood that AA will be made into a pro-inflammatory eicosanoid. The level of that dilution is measured by the AA/EPA ratio.

My Odyssey in Eicosanoids

Remember, my concept of the Zone started when the 1982 Nobel Prize in Medicine was awarded for discoveries of the importance of eicosanoids in chronic disease. This was my "ah-ha" moment. At the time, I was doing research in intravenous drug delivery technology for cancer drugs, using a specialized group of fats known as phospholipids. Because eicosanoids are derived from dietary fats, I had been following eicosanoid research for several years alongside my own research in phospholipids. But after the 1982 Nobel Prize, I quickly realized that I could apply the principles of intravenous drug delivery technology to food in order to induce the body to make more good eicosanoids and fewer bad eicosanoids. If successful, this would result in the equivalent of the holy grail for not only treating chronic disease by controlling silent inflammation but also increasing the cellular rejuvenation potential of every one of the body's 100 trillion cells and reversing many of the chronic disease conditions associated with Toxic Fat Syndrome while improving anti-aging potential at the same time. It couldn't get any better than that.

The science behind eicosanoids is complex (see appendix D), but here is the short version. The overproduction of bad eicosanoids causes the rapid development of chronic disease, whereas increasing the levels of good eicosanoids will increase cellular rejuvenation in every organ. By improving the balance of good and bad eicosanoids, we will live longer and better.

My First Attempts

As early as 1982, I thought reducing AA levels would be relatively easy. Just build up dihomo-gamma-linolenic acid (DGLA) levels by adding more of its immediate precursor (GLA) to the diet, and then add enough EPA to block the enzyme (delta-5-desaturase) that would otherwise continue to convert DGLA into AA at the same time. Remember, good eicosanoids come from DGLA while bad eicosanoids are derived from AA.

Getting EPA was pretty easy: just obtain some fish oil. (Little did I realize how poor the quality of fish oil was back then.) The difficult part was how to increase DGLA levels—the building block of good eicosanoids—at the same time. Theoretically, all I would need is a reliable source of its immediate precursor, GLA, to add to the fish oil to be sure to make adequate levels of DGLA.

I reasoned if just enough GLA could be added to the diet, it would be rapidly converted to DGLA. Then by adding enough fish oil to help block the conversion of DGLA to AA, it should tilt the AA/DGLA ratio to automatically start making more good eicosanoids and fewer bad ones, simply by changing the balance of these two omega-6 fatty acids in every cell in the body, in essence, playing a biochemical lottery in each of the 100 trillion cells. By lowering AA and raising DGLA in each cell's membranes, the chances increased that any eicosanoid made would more likely be a good one (anti-inflammatory) than a bad one (pro-inflammatory). No drug could do that, but maybe the right combination of fatty acids could.

The beginning of my eicosanoid odyssey was to find a suitable seed source rich in GLA, which first led me to the bowels of the MIT library where I found that only about fifty plants in the world contained any GLA. Of those fifty, only five had any significant amounts of GLA. I contacted scientists at Purdue University to see which of the five remaining seeds had the greatest potential for large-scale cultivation. The choice was narrowed down to one seed: borage. So far so good.

Unfortunately, it turned out that all the borage seeds in the world at that time could be packed into the corner of a very small room. After convincing my brother, Doug, to join me in this quest to corner the world's borage market in 1983, we started buying every seed available. We succeeded, because the entire world's supply was pretty limited. Now that Doug and I had cornered the borage seed market, the only trouble was that no one knew how to grow these seeds on a large industrial scale.

We had two options based on where the borage appeared to grow best—the upper plains of Saskatchewan in Canada or the valleys of lower New Zealand. Canada was closer, so Doug and I spent the next year working with selected farmers in that province to develop a crop that had never before existed. By 1984, we were ready to change the world.

GLA: Powerful But Potentially Dangerous

I knew early on that there was a potential problem using GLA: its ability to increase AA levels and thus increase silent inflammation. But I figured if I used enough of the existing types of fish oil, the levels of EPA might be sufficient to stop the spillover of any added GLA into increased production of AA (your worst nightmare). Not surprisingly, I called this the "spillover effect."

So what better way to try out a theory than by human experimentation. My brother and I used ourselves as human guinea pigs, and after going through a number of different combinations of fish oil and borage oil, we came up with a ratio that we thought would work for everyone. Unfortunately, life is never that simple. It might have been a good ratio for the Sears brothers, but not everyone in the world had the same genetics as Doug and me (my wife being a prime example). I experimented with different combinations of EPA and GLA, tried different cycling approaches, and eventually developed different compositions for men and women. The end result was I had to fine-tune the right dose on an individual basis. When it worked, it worked great. But it certainly didn't lend itself to mass marketing, where one size has to fit all. Nonetheless, we kept plowing ahead, primarily using elite athletes as our test subjects although we were really developing this dietary approach for the treatment of chronic diseases such as heart disease. (This was a pretty important reason for my brother and me since everyone on the male side of our family had died from premature heart disease.)

The reason elite athletes are great test subjects is they are often willing to try things for the sake of increased performance. More importantly, they could handle any potential side effects better than diabetic or cardiovascular patients.

Starting first with professional triathletes, then with the Los Angeles Rams (this shows how long ago I was working on this), then the Stanford University swim teams, and finally with numerous Olympic athletes, the end result was always the same: dramatic increases in performance and equally spectacular decreases in recovery times. These were the types of benefits usually provided by anabolic steroids. The right combination of EPA and GLA allowed them to train harder, recover faster, and perform better. It gave them a powerful competitive advantage—yet one that was completely legal and healthy. All these benefits were from decreases in silent inflammation coupled with an increase of the body's internal anti-inflammatory responses that came simply from making more good eicosanoids (from DGLA) and fewer bad ones (from AA).

The downside of this beautiful theory on eicosanoid modification was that the right dosage had to be fine-tuned for each athlete. So we began cycling the athletes, going from a low GLA dose to a higher one and back down again (just like anabolic steroids) to try to prevent the spillover effect. It was time-consuming, but what else could we do?

It turns out that EPA was not as good an inhibitor of delta-5-desaturase enzyme as I originally thought. Although it does have a slight inhibitory effect on AA production, it is not nearly as great as the reduction of insulin levels. This explains why when you add high amounts of EPA and docosahexaenoic acid (DHA) to humans, the levels of these omega-3 fatty acids can be dramatically increased in the blood while only slightly decreasing AA levels. The primary benefits of EPA is dilution of the concentration of AA in the membrane, thus decreasing its likelihood of being made into a bad eicosanoid.

Because of this dilution effect of EPA, when the cell calls out for an eicosanoid and plucks out an appropriate fatty acid from the membrane, it will more likely be EPA than AA. This increases the likelihood of making a relatively neutral eicosanoid (from EPA) as opposed to a powerful pro-inflammatory one (from AA).

The ideal situation, however, is to replace AA with more DGLA so you can increase the potential of making powerful anti-inflammatory eicosanoids. Theoretically this can be done by finding better inhibitors of the enzyme that converts DGLA into AA, thus building up even higher levels of DGLA by adding more GLA to the diet.

The Dynamics of the Spillover Effect

This is what makes GLA so tricky in the wrong hands (like the sales clerk behind the counter at the local health-food store). Initially, when you supplement the diet with GLA, DGLA levels will increase, and you begin making more good eicosanoids. Everything just keeps getting better and better. But at some point, depending on the person's genetics and diet, more of the surplus DGLA gets converted into AA. It turns out that even the doses of fish oil I was providing gave only partial inhibition of the activity of the key enzyme that converts DGLA into AA so that with time, more AA was made. In some people, it never happened, in others it took months, and in some (like my wife) it took only a matter of days.

The Role of the Zone Diet

Once I realized the importance of controlling insulin, I had to go back to the drawing board to develop a dietary program that could also control insulin. The program came to be known as the Zone Diet. It's creation was an effort on my part to control this spillover effect of DGLA into AA. By controlling the levels of insulin through the Zone Diet, the activity of the delta-5-desaturase enzyme could be inhibited to a much greater extent than with EPA alone, thus reducing the flow of DGLA into AA. Once I incorporated the Zone Diet into my overall eicosanoid control dietary program in 1991, I was vastly more successful in using combinations of standard fish oil and borage oil to control the balance of good and bad eicosanoids.

High-Dose EPA/DHA Concentrates: A Potentially Better Solution

The continuing challenge of adding the right amount of fish oil to the right amount of GLA, even with strict adherence to the Zone Diet, was still a very big stumbling block to my initial vision to change the world of medicine simply by changing the balance of good and bad eicosanoids. Frankly, it still required too much thinking for the average person.

Maybe the problem was I simply wasn't using enough EPA to block the formation of AA. Unfortunately, even the best fish oil that I had to work with at the time was frankly pretty bad stuff. It wasn't very rich in EPA, and it also contained a lot of toxins, such as mercury, PCBs, and dioxins. So adding more of this type of fish oil made very little sense.

I became very excited when the first generation of highly concentrated preparations containing high levels of EPA was developed around the year 2000. As I explain in appendix E, these new fish oils were essentially "weapons-grade" fish oil: far more potent and far more purified. Now maybe I could give enough of these purified EPA/DHA concentrates to block the excess formation of AA sufficiently so I could decrease silent inflammation while simultaneously increasing DGLA levels. This would completely eliminate the need for adding any GLA and hence eliminate any problems with the spillover effect.

By this time I was doing a lot of blood testing to determine with precision the levels of these fatty acids in the blood. I knew that if I could reduce the AA/EPA ratio in the blood, this would be the key to reversing Toxic Fat Syndrome, as well as determining the ideal dosage of these EPA/DHA concentrates. This led me into the world of high-dose EPA/DHA concentrates.

Every fish oil researcher I initially contacted about using high doses of these new EPA/DHA concentrates said people would either start bleeding to death, have their immune systems shut down, or show other adverse reactions if I gave them the doses I was proposing, although I now had a blood test to monitor the dosage. (Of course, at the same time, they were also really interested to see if it worked—as long as I would be responsible for all the blame if it didn't work out!) I figured what was needed was a clinical guideline of how much of these new EPA/DHA concentrates I could safely give to a person to make sure that none of these apocalyptic events would happen.

Even in the late 1990s, there was very little published research on what an optimal dose might be. Basically, a researcher would simply guess. I decided that rather than guessing, I would start from the opposite direction—determine the AA/EPA ratio in the healthiest people on earth and add enough of these new EPA/DHA concentrates to reach the same ratio. The Japanese were the longest-lived people in the world with the greatest health span, besides having the lowest rates of heart disease and depression, so I figured they would be pretty good candidates to determine what the ideal AA/EPA ratio should be in the blood.

It turns out the average AA/EPA ratio in the Japanese population was between 1.5 and 3.

Because the Japanese weren't bleeding to death (even though they take aspirin) or rapidly dying of infectious disease, I believed if I could maintain the AA/EPA ratio above 1.5, I would have an excellent safety net. Because I could now measure the AA/EPA ratio, the optimal dosage would be easy to determine.

What I wasn't prepared for were the massive amounts of these new EPA/DHA concentrates that I needed to give to get the blood levels of the typical American anywhere near those of the Japanese. By 2002, I had completed enough research with these high doses of EPA/DHA to publish my first results in my book, *The OmegaRx Zone*.

The wild card was the Zone Diet because of its ability to control AA levels. The more closely a person followed the Zone Diet, the less of these ultra-refined EPA/DHA concentrates they would need to reduce their AA/EPA ratio to one similar to the Japanese. Of course, the less they followed the Zone Diet, the more of the EPA/DHA concentrates they would need to reduce their levels of silent inflammation. It seemed like a pretty fair trade-off at the time because I didn't have to worry about the spillover effect coming from adding extra GLA.

The best example of the benefits of high-dose EPA/DHA concentrates came from the Sago mine disaster in West Virginia in early 2006. Thirteen miners were trapped underground for forty-one hours in a carbon monoxide atmosphere. When the rescue workers finally reached them, only one of the thirteen was alive, and just barely. Randall McCloy was brought out of the mineshaft with brain failure, heart failure, liver failure, and kidney failure. His chances for survival were slim, and if he did live, he would likely end up in a vegetative state of life.

A week after his rescue, his neurosurgeon, Julian Bailes, called me. He wanted to use omega-3 fatty acid supplementation with Randall, but he didn't know much. I told Julian that he would probably have to use about 15 grams of eicosapentaenoic acid (EPA) and docosahexaenoic acid (DHA) per day, coming from these new concentrates. His first response was that I must be kidding. I assured him that I had never had any problems with those doses and immediately air-shipped several bottles to the hospital. For the next two months, Randall received about 15 grams of EPA and DHA per day through his feeding tube. Furthermore, we constantly tested his AA/EPA ratio in the blood on a weekly basis because this was a very extreme case. At no time did his AA/EPA ratio ever go below 3.

At the end of two months, Randall came out of his coma. Two months after that, with continued oral dosing with the same levels of EPA and DHA, he went home with normal heart function, normal liver function, and normal kidney function. Upon arriving home, he gave a short speech to the press worthy of any politician. Medical editors were calling his recovery a "miracle." The only miracle was that Julian trusted my insight into the amounts of EPA and DHA that were needed to reduce high levels of inflammation throughout Randall's body caused by the carbon monoxide poisoning.

In the spring of 2007, Randall and his wife had a healthy child. This was a pretty good indication that everything is now working pretty well.

How Much Do You Need?

This has always been the big question. Now using the AA/EPA ratio in the blood as a reliable clinical marker, it is possible to give a much more defined answer about the amount of ultra-refined EPA/DHA concentrates that are needed to reduce silent inflammation to the levels found in the Japanese population. I quickly found that there was no relationship to age, weight, or gender and the amount of EPA/DHA concentrates required to reduce the levels of silent inflammation. The amount needed depends on the levels of existing silent inflammation, and where in the body it is located. After doing thousands of blood tests, I can give you some rough estimates of the amounts of EPA and DHA you will need on a daily basis to keep silent inflammation under control and begin reversing the clinical consequences of Toxic Fat Syndrome.

Condition	Amount Required
No chronic disease	2.5 grams of EPA and DHA per day
Overweight, obese, type 2 diabetes, heart disease, and before starting any type of weight-loss program	5 grams of EPA and DHA per day
Chronic pain	7.5 grams of EPA and DHA per day
Neurological disorders	10 grams of EPA and DHA per day

If you are normal weight and not inflamed (a very small percentage of Americans, according to my blood testing), then you will probably only need about 2.5 grams of EPA and DHA to reduce your levels of silent inflammation to that found in the Japanese population. This is the amount of EPA and DHA that your parents would have gotten from your grandparents when they had to take a tablespoon of cod-liver oil (probably the world's most disgusting tasting food) every morning before they left the house.

If you are overweight or obese, you already have high levels of AA stored in your adipose tissue, so you will need higher levels of these omega-3 fatty acids to reduce the inflammation in that organ. Keep in mind when you start any diet, you will begin releasing stored AA in the fat cells directly into the bloodstream as you lose weight. Adding back sufficient levels of fish oil will help reduce the negative consequences, due to the transient increase of toxic fat in the bloodstream.

If you have significant clinical consequences (type 2 diabetes or some indication of existing cardiovascular disease) due to long-term exposure to Toxic Fat Syndrome, you will also need more EPA and DHA.

If you have chronic pain ("screaming" inflammation), then the amounts of EPA and DHA required will be even higher (about 7.5 grams of EPA and DHA per day).

Finally, if you have a neurological condition (depression, attention deficit disorder, multiple sclerosis, Alzheimer's, and so on), then be prepared to take more than 10 grams of EPA and DHA per day.

The first thing you are probably thinking is, *Yikes, that's a lot.* But it indicates the severity of existing levels of Toxic Fat Syndrome in Americans due to the Perfect Nutritional Storm. It's also why you need to have very pure EPA/DHA concentrates—because these levels will probably be needed for a lifetime to keep the silent inflammation under control.

How can you tell if the fish oil you are taking is free from contaminants?

The vast majority of all fish oils on the market today come from small fish, such as sardines and anchovies. Even so, the crude fish oil is still heavily contaminated by man-made toxins. The easiest way to tell whether your fish oil is reasonably free from these contaminants is through smell and taste. A very fishy taste or smell of fish oil is highly indicative of oil that has not been sufficiently refined. Much of that taste and smell comes from the presence of breakdown products of the fatty acids known as aldehydes. These are chemicals that are known to cause damage to DNA.

If you want more quantification, then go to www.ifosprogram.com, which is a free site run by the University of Guelph in Ontario. The IFOS (International Fish Oil Standards) program uses the most sophisticated instrumentation to determine the purity of fish oils. Look for those oils with a five-star rating, indicating they are pure, potent, and ready for action.

Let me give you an example of why you may need to take high-dose EPA/DHA concentrates for a lifetime. I published a study in 2007 treating children with attention deficit hyperactivity disorder (ADHD) using high-dose EPA/DHA concentrates. It has long been known that such children have very high AA/EPA ratios in their blood. In our eight-week study we started the children at 15 grams of EPA and DHA per day and then checked their blood levels at four and eight weeks. Even with these high doses, the average AA/EPA ratio at the end of the study was still about 2.5. (This was the same dosage given to Randall McCloy, the surviving Sago miner, and his AA/EPA ratio never dropped below 3.) With this reduction in the AA/EPA ratio came a striking improvement in the children's behavior, judged by their psychiatrist. How long did it take to see improvements in their behavior? About four weeks. How long did it take for the behavior benefits to disappear after they stopped taking the fish oil? About four weeks. So if you want to treat ADHD effectively, you have to take high-dose EPA and DHA for a long time.

How to Take Liquid Fish Oil

Once you make a decision to purchase enough fish oil to have a therapeutic effect, the next question is how to take it. If you need only small amounts (2.5 grams of EPA and DHA per day), then taking four one-gram capsules of ultra-refined EPA/DHA concentrate will be your best choice. However, if you need more EPA and DHA, you should consider taking liquid fish oil. I have found that the upper limit for capsule consumption is usually about four per day of anything. If you are planning to use liquid fish oil, always keep it in the freezer to prevent oxidation and to improve the taste. If it's really good stuff, it won't freeze. Of course, if it does become solid in the freezer, that's a good indication that it may have lots of impurities that have not been removed.

If you are using liquid fish oil, let me tell you some of the tricks I have developed over the years.

The Citrus Trick

One of the oldest tricks is to suck on a slice of citrus fruit (lime, lemon, or even orange) for five seconds before taking the liquid fish oil. The acidity of the citrus fruit (especially lime) will dampen the receptors in your taste buds, so you won't taste the fish oil. (Keep in mind the higher the purity of the fish oil, the better the taste.) Alternatively, mix a little citrus juice (about one ounce) with the fish oil and swig the combination down quickly.

The Fish Oil Shooter

A much better alternative to citrus juice is a polyphenol supplement. Polyphenols are the chemicals that give fruits and vegetables their colors—and are powerful antioxidants that can protect the EPA and DHA from oxidation. Mix one ounce of a suitable liquid polyphenol supplement with liquid fish oil in a tequila glass and throw it back like taking a tequila sunrise cocktail. Just make sure the liquid fish oil is coming directly from the freezer and the polyphenol supplement is refrigerated. It will taste a lot better than using citrus juice. For a change of pace, add one ounce of extra virgin olive oil to the shooter to further dilute the fish oil taste.

The best time to take fish oil is right after a meal, when it will be more readily digested and absorbed. I find that taking it right after the evening meal is the perfect way to decrease the late-night munchies since the EPA in the fish oil will inhibit the binding of endocannabinoids to their receptors in the brain for the next four to six hours.

The Problem with EPA/DHA Concentrates

I was pretty proud that I could use these new high-dose EPA/DHA concentrates alone to reduce silent inflammation. The reduction of the AA/EPA ratio in the blood indicated that I could control pro-inflammatory eicosanoids with remarkable precision. By 2005, when I was beginning to complete a number of clinical studies done by my nonprofit foundation, I could begin to look more closely at the raw data coming from the blood testing. They all indicated that the levels of DGLA were decreasing, not increasing.

The good news was that silent inflammation (as measured by the AA/EPA ratio) could be reduced. The bad news was that the body's internal cellular rejuvenation potential (as measured by the AA/DGLA ratio) was also being reduced. In essence, the body was getting only about 50 percent of the full potential benefits of modifying the balance of good and bad eicosanoids. It was like taking two steps forward and one step backward.

Back to the Future

I figured that half a loaf (using only high-dose EPA/DHA concentrates without any added GLA) was better than none. But I still wanted to get the whole enchilada of decreasing pro-inflammation while simultaneously increasing the body's own internal anti-inflammatory responses that lead to continual cellular rejuvenation and ultimate wellness for a lifetime—the true definition of anti-aging.

The answer to this dilemma rested on finding better inhibitors of the delta-5-desaturase enzyme than EPA. If you could find this type of inhibitor, you could now safely add back GLA that would be rapidly metabolized into DGLA, but this new inhibitor would prevent the spillover effect of the further metabolism of DGLA into AA. The end result would dramatically improve the already robust benefits of high-dose

EPA/DHA concentrates. The answer was found back in my kitchen: toasted sesame oil.

Sesame oil has been used for thousands of years as a cooking oil. It has also been known that when the seeds are toasted before the extraction of the oil, the resulting oil is much more stable and seems to have a lot more health benefits. Now we understand why. Although sesame oil is rich in omega-6 fatty acids, it also contains a very small percentage of compounds known as lignans. These sesame lignans are very special because they are specific inhibitors of the delta-5-desaturase enzyme that converts DGLA to AA.

But the most powerful inhibitor of this enzyme turns out to be a thermal breakdown product of the lignans, made when the seeds are toasted before the extraction of the oil. That breakdown product is called *sesamol*.

Here was the key to finally making super fish oils that could simultaneously decrease silent inflammation and increase the body's internal anti-inflammatory response. By combining high levels of EPA (using EPA/DHA concentrates) to reduce silent inflammation with the correct amount of GLA and just the right amount of toasted sesame oil concentrate to increase the body's internal cellular rejuvenation potential, you would have the answer. This is why I call it super fish oil. It is kind of like making a complex sauce for a five-star restaurant.

The end result of using such a "super" fish oil is that each cell in the body is able to make more good eicosanoids and fewer bad ones. This was exactly what I was trying to achieve when my brother and I headed twenty-five years earlier to the frozen prairies of Saskatchewan.

With these new super fish oils, it is no longer simply a matter of reducing the levels of a toxic fat (AA) but of simultaneously creating high levels of a great fat (DGLA).

Summary

Trying to navigate through all the numerous fish oil products is confusing at best. Furthermore, the amount you need is not dependent on your age, weight, or sex, but it does depend on your levels of silent inflammation and where it is located. This means most Americans are going to need a lot. However, taking fish oil alone inhibits the formation of DGLA, thus reducing the body's cellular rejuvenation potential. Trying to compensate by adding GLA is a very tricky proposition. The final key is adding toasted sesame oil concentrate and GLA in the correct ratio, allowing you to maintain the ideal balance of DGLA, AA, and EPA with the grand prize of a lifelong control of silent inflammation along with an increase in the body's own internal anti-inflammatory responses, which are needed for a longer and better life.

CHAPTER 10

Putting It All Together

I N THE LAST TWO CHAPTERS, I GAVE YOU ALL THE DIETARY TOOLS you need to reverse Toxic Fat Syndrome and combat silent inflammation for a lifetime. Now you just have to put them all together.

In essence, you are trying to orchestrate three rather complex tasks simultaneously:

➤ Reducing the intake of calories by changing the balance of hormones that control both satiety and hunger in the brain

➤ Reducing insulin levels by controlling the balance of protein to the glycemic load of a meal

➤ Reducing the production of arachidonic acid (AA) by reducing the intake of omega-6 fats while increasing the consumption of long-chain omega-3 fats, such as eicosapentaenoic acid (EPA) and docosahexaenoic acid (DHA)

It sounds pretty complex. Actually, the events happening inside your body *are* complex, but all you have to do is follow the Zone Diet and take adequate levels of fish oil on a consistent basis. If you do these two things, you will reverse Toxic Fat Syndrome and live a longer and better life.

Blame It on Your Genes

No one wants to become overweight or obese, let alone develop heart disease, cancer, or Alzheimer's. The health problems that presently confront us are multi-factorial, with many different genes interacting negatively with our current dietary environment to maintain constantly high levels of silent inflammation. You can't change your genes, but you can change their expression and optimize your health, simply by eating smart. You can think of the foods you eat like a medicine to be taken at the right dose and at the right time—but much better tasting, of course.

Convergence of Genomics and Nutrition

The primary cause of our continuing crisis of America's health-care system is the growing disconnect between our genes and our diets. New studies indicate that aging Americans who are ready to retire and are close to Medicare age are far less healthy than their predecessors some forty to fifty years ago. The lead author of that study, Beth Soldo of the University of Pennsylvania, pointed out, "It's not what I expected." The implications of a growing wave of increasingly unhealthy baby boomers gaining virtually unlimited, free (at least for them) health-care benefits when they turn sixty-five is a fiscally frightening thought.

Why have the promises of drugs (let alone the promises of the supplement industry) let us down? The answer is both simple and complex: genetics. Drugs are based on the one-disease, one-drug approach. That's great for bacterial infections, but not for obesity, diabetes, heart disease, cancer, and Alzheimer's. These are diseases caused by the spread of silent inflammation to other organs in the body. This is the result of the interaction of our current pro-inflammatory diet with a wide variety of our genes, especially those that affect inflammation.

Recent advances in molecular biology are now providing the insight into how the food we eat is causing the genetic expression of inflammatory genes. This is called *nutrigenomics* (see appendix G). But in essence, nutrigenomics is how the correct use of our diet may be the "miracle" drug we are searching for to reduce silent inflammation for a lifetime.

Simply stated, the Zone Diet can turn genes off that promote silent inflammation as well as turn genes on that promote cellular rejuvenation. That's a pretty powerful statement. Once you understand the implications of that, it begins to elevate nutrition to a much higher level in the pecking order of health-care interventions.

In many ways, our current health problems (obesity and chronic disease) can be viewed as a mismatch between our genes and an increasingly pro-inflammatory diet to which those genes are exposed. The end result has been the rise in silent inflammation that drives Toxic Fat Syndrome with the consequences of increased obesity, more rapid development of chronic diseases, and faster aging. You can't change your genes, but you definitely can change their expression using the

Zone Diet. Thus the Zone Diet can be viewed as a way of life (that is, diet) to alter the expression of your genes, especially those that deal with silent inflammation. That is something you have to follow for a lifetime to squeeze the most out of your genes.

Diet-induced responses can activate the most elementary part of our immune system, which is the mainstay of our immunological defense system—our innate immune system. Many of the components of the innate immune system in plants are virtually identical to humans. It is only recently with the advent of the new tools of molecular biology that we have come to realize how complex the innate immune system actually is. If this part of your immune system is activated by something you eat, then your inflammatory response is constantly turned on, thus accelerating the development of chronic disease and aging. Ultimately, your levels of silent inflammation are controlled by what you eat and how the various components of your diet interact with the innate immune system. (See appendix G for more details.) However, this also means you have the potential to modulate the innate immune system by following the Zone Wellness Pyramid.

The Zone Wellness Pyramid

Nutrition has always been considered as the poor relation of drugs (at least for the last seventy years). Those who could prescribe drugs were considered to be the masters of the universe. What you ate didn't matter as long as you took your medications. The end result of this mentality is a health system that is rapidly breaking down. We spend more on health care than any other country in the world, and we don't have a lot to show for it. I believe this is because we have neglected the basic foundation of our health—what we eat.

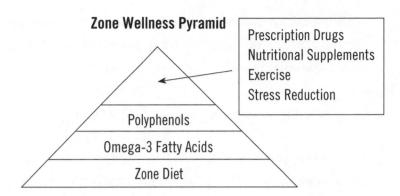

Zone Wellness Pyramid

Prescription Drugs
Nutritional Supplements
Exercise
Stress Reduction

Polyphenols

Omega-3 Fatty Acids

Zone Diet

Consider your diet as a foundation for controlling silent inflammation, which translates into increased wellness. It's like building a house. You can build it on a concrete foundation or on sand. Which of the two houses will have the greater longevity? The same is true for your body. Whatever you are doing to maintain your state of wellness (building the house)—whether it is exercise, prescription drugs (including hormone replacement therapy), nutritional supplements, and even meditation—won't work unless you have a sound dietary foundation to build upon.

But if your dietary foundation is unsound, no matter how expensive the drug or how diligently you follow a lifestyle intervention, the end results will never reach their expected potential. How often do you hear a physician say, "That drug should have worked. Oh well, let's try another," or know someone who exercises daily for hours but doesn't seem to drop a pound? All the potential benefits of the drug or exercise are being undermined by a poor dietary foundation that increases silent inflammation, so you are constantly running uphill in order to maintain wellness.

What if you had a dietary foundation that decreased silent inflammation by turning *off* pro-inflammatory genes while simultaneously turning *on* anti-inflammatory ones? Then the outcome is very different.

You get great, consistent results with the least amount of effort. That's the promise of building upon an anti-inflammatory diet based on the Zone Wellness Pyramid.

The Zone Diet: The Foundation of Wellness

The first and most important tier of the Zone Wellness Pyramid consists of the Zone Diet. The power of the Zone Diet lies in its ability to reduce AA levels. If you reduce AA levels, Toxic Fat Syndrome begins to recede. The purpose of the Zone Diet is to balance the hormones (insulin, glucagon, and eicosanoids) that are influencing your inflammatory response. Too low of an inflammatory response makes it difficult to ward off microbial invaders or repair injuries. On the other hand, too high of an inflammatory response begins attacking every cell in your body. You want to maintain your inflammatory responses in a therapeutic zone.

The Zone Diet is a way of life to reduce, if not reverse, the consequences of Toxic Fat Syndrome. While it can be a quick "fix" with beneficial results in as little as three days, it's really a clinically validated way of controlling silent inflammation for a lifetime.

This also means you have to do some thinking because the balance of your hormones is only as good as your last meal, and will only be as good as your next meal. Controlling Toxic Fat Syndrome ultimately means keeping your hormones in a zone throughout the day. To achieve this, you want to try to make each meal as close to Zone parameters as possible: one-third low-fat protein, two-thirds colorful carbohydrates (primarily vegetables, limited amounts of fruits, and using grains and starches as condiments), and a dash of heart-healthy monounsaturated fat (olive oil, slivered almonds, and even guacamole).

Omega-3 Fatty Acids: Your Safety Net Against Silent Inflammation

The second tier of the Zone Wellness Pyramid is consuming adequate levels of omega-3 fatty acids rich in EPA and DHA, which are also powerful inhibitors of several stages of the activation of our more primitive inflammatory responses. The omega-3 fatty acids will not decrease AA levels as much as the Zone Diet, but by increasing the levels of EPA, you dilute the likelihood of AA being plucked from the cell membrane to be transformed into a pro-inflammatory eicosanoid. You can view this as further reinforcements to protect against silent inflammation. But omega-3 fatty acids have more benefits than simply diluting excess AA. They can also alter membrane fluidity, modulate ion channels in cells, and affect genetic expression.

Let me emphasize again the word *sufficient*. As I pointed out in the previous chapter, this is going to be a lot of EPA and DHA for most Americans. This just indicates how inflamed Americans are. The good news is that it only takes fifteen seconds a day to take enough EPA and DHA to address the situation. To further improve the benefits of supplemental EPA and DHA, consider taking super fish oils to ensure that you are not decreasing your body's internal cellular rejuvenation potential.

Polyphenols: Getting Color into Your Diet

The third dietary tier of the Zone Wellness Pyramid is consuming adequate levels of dietary polyphenols. These are the chemicals in fruits and vegetables that provide color. At high enough concentrations, these plant chemicals have anti-inflammatory benefits as well as activate other key enzymes that lead to increased ATP production in the body.

This is why the Zone Diet is also rich in fruits and vegetables—these are the carbohydrates that are rich in polyphenols. It's also why grains and starches are used in moderation on the diet. (Remember: no color, no polyphenols.)

Before 1995, there was very little written on polyphenols. Through advances in molecular biology, we now know they are one of the few anti-inflammatory defense mechanisms that plants have against microbial invaders. There are more than eight thousand known polyphenols, and perhaps three times that amount that have not yet been chemically identified. With so many polyphenols, it is obvious that no single one polyphenol has a unique magical power, as many health-food marketers would lead you to believe.

If you are following the Zone Diet precisely, you are getting about ten to fifteen servings of fruits and vegetables per day. That amount of vegetables and fruits means you are also getting a lot of anti-inflammatory polyphenols. By eating a broad spectrum of colorful vegetables and fruits, you are also getting a broad range of polyphenols to effectively inhibit silent inflammation. This is why your grandmother told you that you couldn't leave the table until you had eaten all your vegetables. Who knew she was on the cutting edge of molecular biology?

All the Other Stuff We Do and Buy

The final part of the Zone Wellness Pyramid includes all the things we have been led to believe are the "real" foundation of wellness. These include prescription drugs, nutritional supplements, exercise, and stress reduction. These can have benefits, but if a strong dietary foundation is not present, they will have far less effect on your future wellness than you might anticipate.

Whatever you want out of life—weight loss, longevity, improved health, better mental and physical performance as well as better emotional control—can be controlled by hormones that can be orchestrated by lifelong adherence to the Zone Wellness Pyramid.

Less Than 30 Days to Begin Reversing Toxic Fat Syndrome

Let's be frank, virtually everyone in America has some level of Toxic Fat Syndrome. Don't despair. It takes less than thirty days to begin reversing it. Follow the Zone Wellness Pyramid, and you have a clinically proven pathway to begin reversing Toxic Fat Syndrome in less than thirty days. That's the good news. But remember, you have to continue this anti-inflammatory way of eating for the rest of your life if you don't want Toxic Fat Syndrome to reappear.

Time: Your Greatest Enemy

Reversing Toxic Fat Syndrome is easy if you are willing to make the time to do it. And here is the problem: time. Rather than give you dietary advice that simply won't be followed in the real world, I have found it more productive to provide different dietary prescriptions all depending on the amount of time a person is willing to devote to keeping silent inflammation under control on a lifetime basis.

The Fifteen-Second Prescription

This is the Zone prescription that most people are interested in because fifteen seconds a day is all they are usually willing to expend to maintain their wellness. If this is your maximum time allotment, then simply consume as much ultra-refined EPA/DHA concentrate as you need in less than fifteen seconds, and call it a day. With that one simple action, you have gone a great distance to reduce silent inflammation, by diluting out toxic fat, and to move to a higher state of wellness in thirty days. This is what happened to Randall McCloy (the sole survivor of the Sago mine disaster), and it can happen to you. If fish oil happens to be super fish oil, you get the added benefit of increasing cellular rejuvenation (that is, anti-aging) in each of your 100 trillion cells.

The amount of fish oil you need for the fifteen-second prescription doesn't depend on your age, weight, or sex, but it does depend on how much silent inflammation you have and where it is located, as discussed in the previous chapter.

My recommendations for EPA and DHA require taking a lot of fish oil. And here's the problem with natural products: they can work very effectively, but you have to take a lot to see a therapeutic benefit. If you take a small dose, then you get little, if any, positive effects. The second thing you should notice is my recommendations are based on the grams of EPA and DHA, not the amount of fish oil itself. People often don't realize that most of the fatty acids in a typical fish oil supplement are not EPA and DHA. In fact, in most fish oil products, the levels of EPA and DHA constitute only a small proportion of the total fat content. The amounts of EPA and DHA in fish oil can vary from as low as 15 percent (as in cod-liver oil) to over 60 percent (as in ultra-refined EPA/DHA concentrates). Most fish oils you find in health-food stores are at about 30 percent. The lower the amount of EPA and DHA, the greater the amount of total fish oil you have to consume to get a therapeutic effect.

Surprisingly, if you actually calculate the price of EPA and DHA per gram of fish oil, some of the highly purified fish oils are actually less expensive than what you find in Wal-Mart. How is this possible? Less purified fish oil is less expensive, but the soft gelatin capsule used to encapsulate it is not. Often the cost of the capsule is ten times the cost of the fish oil inside of it. This is just another case of buyer beware. To add insult to injury, these less refined fish oils are the ones that give the burping, fishy aftertaste, and other gastric complaints that make long-term compliance unlikely.

The Five-Minute Prescription

People who can handle the fifteen-second prescription may be willing to try the five-minute prescription. In this case, you simply replace one meal per day with a prepared Zone meal replacement that has the right balance of protein, low glycemic-load carbohydrates, and fat (think of the 1-2-3 rule). However, the meal replacement needs to taste great in addition to being convenient, affordable, and portable (so you can eat it in a car or walking down the street). But most importantly, it has to suppress hunger for at least four, and ideally six, hours.

To test the feasibility of this approach, I experimented with obese patients who were considering gastric bypass surgery. Before they were scheduled to go under the knife, they were offered the opportunity to try replacing all of their meals for thirty days with Zone meal replacements as well as supplementing their diets with high-dose EPA/DHA concentrates (5 grams of EPA and DHA per day). The average results:

Parameter	Start	30 Days	% Change
Weight	229	219	-4
BMI	37.7	36.1	-4
Total Cholesterol	203	177	-13
Triglycerides (TG)	232	177	-24

Parameter	Start	30 Days	% Change
TG/HDL	4.2	2.6	-38
AA/EPA	22	7	-68

Although the individuals lost only an average of about ten pounds of weight each during this four-week period and were still considered severely obese (BMI > 35), they were elated about the changes in their blood chemistry and, more important, how they felt. In fact, they were feeling so good that they all canceled their scheduled surgeries. Essentially, they had gone from having a malignant adipose tumor to a benign adipose tumor in thirty days. Their total time commitment was about fifteen minutes (three Zone meal replacements at five minutes each) plus another fifteen seconds to consume a therapeutic amount of EPA and DHA every day. The patients following this Zone program were getting the same clinical benefits from this thirty-day dietary program, without the wide variety of side effects that comes with gastric bypass surgery (death is one) as well as not facing the need for several additional cosmetic surgeries that often are needed after the initial surgery.

The Thirty-Minute Prescription

Meal replacements are never meant to be used on lifetime basis. That's why you want to be making your own Zone meals. Unfortunately, time remains your enemy. It takes time to get the ingredients, prepare them, and cook the meals. Most of the meals in the twenty-eight-day meal plans in this book take less than thirty minutes to prepare. Rather than going into a repeat of my previous books, I recommend picking up *Zone Meals in Seconds* to get all the information you need to make Zone meals anytime and anywhere. Several of my other books rich in

Zone recipes include *Mastering the Zone, Zone Meals in Minutes,* and *The Top 100 Zone Foods.*

The Three-Hour Prescription

This is the ultimate expression of an anti-inflammatory lifestyle because it includes exercise and stress reduction. But it takes more time. You must daily have adequate levels of fish oil (fifteen seconds of your time), prepare three Zone meals, spend thirty to sixty minutes in moderate exercise, and finally, sit in a comfortable chair, thinking of nothing for twenty minutes (this is called stress reduction). These are all "drugs" that have to be taken for a lifetime. The three-hour prescription is the basis for Zone Living. Each element works synergistically with the others to control silent inflammation as well as give you a lifetime of weight maintenance. There is no drug or combination of drugs that can do it, but your diet and your lifestyle can.

Summary

Although the hormonal control mechanisms behind the Zone Diet taking place in your body are complex, incorporating them into your life is easy. You simply choose your level of time commitment. If you only have fifteen extra seconds a day, then take as much fish oil as you can in that fifteen seconds. If you are willing to spend five minutes a day, take your fish oil and replace one meal with a functional food product that meets the 1-2-3 balance that will keep you in the Zone for a four- to six-hour period. If you can spend one and a half hours a day, take your fish oil, and prepare three Zone meals. And for the complete synergistic benefits of Zone Living, take your fish oil, prepare your own Zone meals, do moderate exercise, and practice stress reduction—which adds up to about three hours. It's all a matter of your degree of commitment to keeping silent inflammation under control for a lifetime.

It sounds so low-tech, but what is happening in your body is extremely high-tech as you are now in the process of turning off inflammatory genes and turning on anti-inflammatory genes at the same time. No drug can do that, but your diet can.

CHAPTER 11

Overcoming Obstacles to Your Success

NO ONE PLANS TO BECOME FAT. ALTHOUGH THERE ARE A LOT OF misconceptions about the obesity epidemic, it still remains the greatest threat to our health-care system because it is one of the first signs that silent inflammation already exists in the adipose tissue. If it begins to spread into the bloodstream, then you have Toxic Fat Syndrome. While the dietary pathway to reverse Toxic Fat Syndrome is clear, numerous formidable obstacles stand in your way. Some are technological, others biological, and still others political. The more you know about each, the more likely you can circumvent them in order to make wellness your lifelong companion.

In times of crisis, fingers always start pointing at who is to blame for the rise of obesity. Fast food, television, computer games, and so on are the usual suspects. These explanations might work in America, but they don't work well in other parts of the world, such as Italy, where children were the leanest in Europe a generation ago but are now the fattest. And it also doesn't explain the worldwide explosion in obesity where we now have more overweight than malnourished people on the planet.

The underlying driving forces to explain these phenomena are much more powerful than you are led to believe.

Technology

The primary cause of any seismic change in human behavior is not a person, group, or international consortium. It's technology. The epidemics of obesity and Toxic Fat Syndrome are no different. Through much of mankind's history, producing, transporting, and preparing food has been a major struggle in both time and expense. All of these factors have radically changed. Look at the reduction of the cost of food as a percentage of disposable income. In America we have the cheapest food in the world: only about 10 percent of our disposable income goes to food. Contrast this to Japan, where about 20 percent of disposable income goes to food. Needless to say, the portion sizes in Japan are considerably less than those in America.

Three technological factors have reduced food costs in America. First are the tremendous advances in agribusiness that allow very few people to generate massive amounts of raw materials, and in particular refined carbohydrates and vegetable oils. Second is a transport system that is second to none in efficiently moving raw materials from the site of production to the consumer's kitchen. But the third is the most important: our advanced processed-food technology that allows us to make virtually anything out of cheap grains and vegetable oils with a virtually unlimited shelf life. All of these have contributed to dramatically reduce the cost of food and, more important, the amount of time needed to prepare it.

Sixty years ago most of the world was trying to cope with preventing starvation after World War II. The only highly industrialized country virtually unscathed by the war was the United States. We had the raw materials and the industrial capacity to begin developing what is known as the agribusiness sector. With advanced technology and the consolidation of family farms into giant enterprises, the ability to produce raw materials for processed foods in America became unsurpassed in the world.

All of this was accelerated with changes in farm subsidies as I described earlier. The primary food ingredients that came from this government largess were cheap refined carbohydrates and cheap vegetable oils. From these two food components came a virtually inexhaustible stream of new processed foods, and the impact of the ingredients of those foods began to alter the natural balance of hormones that eventually control our hunger and satiety. But there was an associated cost that no one ever calculated: the rapid rise of Toxic Fat Syndrome. The combination of cheap refined carbohydrates that increase insulin levels coupled with cheap vegetable oils providing large amounts of omega-6 fatty acids is a surefire prescription for increased silent inflammation. It's like adding gasoline to a fire.

Globalization of Food Ingredients

High levels of silent inflammation may be a very recent phenomenon in human history. It can be traced to the introduction of processed foods. This includes not only junk food but also vegetable oil and food products based on refined carbohydrates, such as bread, pasta, and breakfast cereals. Keep in mind that without cheap food ingredients, the processed food industry doesn't make money.

The United States has also become the low-cost producer of the ingredients required to make processed foods. It is far cheaper for Italians to buy corn or soybean oil (both rich in omega-6 fatty acids) made in the Midwest than olive oil made in Italy. Even after shipping expenses, corn or soybean oil undercuts the price of olive oil (virtually devoid in omega-6 fatty acids) by a factor of five.

Today the American processed food industry stands unchallenged as the leader in the world. That's why Toxic Fat Syndrome first appeared in America and is now spreading worldwide as the globalization of processed foods takes a greater and greater percentage of the world food dollar. The cost of processed foods has decreased dramatically with increased technology and government subsidies, increased shelf life, and thus increased ease of distribution. Furthermore, the cost of refined carbohydrates and vegetable oils is about four hundred times cheaper per calorie than fresh fruit and vegetables. It doesn't take an economic genius to understand that given the choice between processed food products that are convenient, cheap (as well as taste great), and last forever and natural foods that are more expensive, difficult to prepare, and likely to go bad, the consumer is going to prefer the former.

Snacking: Freedom to Eat Whatever, Whenever, and with Whomever You Want

Freedom is a very difficult thing to retract once it appears. In the era of cable TV and the Internet, would you ever go back to having only three choices of TV for nightly viewing? Or traveling to work on a bus, if you have your own car? The list goes on. Once you have the freedom of choice, it is hard to put the genie back into the bottle.

The same is true of food. While eating remains a social experience, the dynamics have changed completely. In the old days, the cost of food ingredients was high, and the time to prepare them was long. It made perfect economic sense to have three family meals per day where everyone got together at the same time to eat the same thing. I remember when growing up, if I wanted something different, my mother would constantly tell me, "I am not your short-order cook." Of course, I had my trump card to avoid going hungry if I didn't like what was being served at that meal. I would eat a bowl of Grape-Nuts. It was convenient, it was within my very limited cooking skills, and it tasted great. Grape-Nuts for breakfast, Grape-Nuts when I came home after basketball practice, Grape-Nuts for dinner, and Grape-Nuts as a nighttime snack. In hindsight, I can't think of a worse choice I could have made.

The cooking skills required to eat this new generation of processed foods are virtually zero. Their portability is great as we can take our processed foods anywhere, including in our cars, which are now the new dining rooms for many Americans. Processed foods are extremely palatable, and we can eat with our friends (in food courts at the mall) instead of with our families.

Another issue is variety. As humans, we constantly seek new varieties of the same thing to ensure that it doesn't get boring. To this end, the processed-food industry has the solution—make many varieties of the same thing, such as twenty-four types of Oreos. Same Oreos, but each is a different size, shape, color, or taste to give the impression that we are eating something new instead of the same old repackaged Oreo cookie.

These new freedoms for expanding the social experience of eating whatever, whenever, and with whomever we want mean that the family meal is never coming back again. And because processed foods are available anywhere, if you are constantly hungry, that urge can be satisfied very quickly.

Unexpected Factors

Most obesity experts focus on only two factors to explain the obesity epidemic: consuming too many calories and not getting enough exercise. They consider no other factors that might also explain the rapid increase in obesity. This has been a great mistake because these other factors mean that a simple solution such as "eat less and exercise more" isn't likely to be the answer.

Sugar Addiction

One of the most disturbing side effects of our increasing dependence on cheap carbohydrates with a high glycemic load is that we may be becoming physically addicted to them. This was demonstrated in a 2007 study in France in which cocaine-addicted rats were offered access to super-sweetened water using a combination of an artificial sweetener and sucrose. Within three days, the cocaine-addicted rats switched their allegiance from cocaine to the super-sweetened sugar water. It turns out that glucose can activate dopamine receptors much like cocaine. But unlike cocaine, there are no adverse effects on the sympathetic nervous system. If the rats get a hit of glucose, they gain the effects of cocaine without the downside of increased nervousness. Since cocaine is one of the most addictive substances known, guess what happens when humans get the same hit on their dopamine receptors by constantly eating sugar? They become addicted, and they go into withdrawal if they can't get it quickly. The processed food industry ensures that will never happen.

Sleep Deprivation

One unanticipated consequence of computers has been an increase in sleep deprivation. The number of hours for sleeping is decreasing. Frankly, we have more things (such as surfing the Internet and instant messaging) to keep us up. By staying awake, you build up a sleep debt that has to be paid off sometime. The usual way is taking naps. (This may be why taking naps three times a week can lower your risk of developing heart disease.) But if sleep debt continues, a corresponding hormonal response to this stress occurs: the increased secretion of the hormone cortisol. One consequence of high levels of cortisol is an increase in insulin resistance, leading to elevated insulin levels that drive down blood sugar levels (see appendix F). The easiest (but most dangerous) way to address low blood sugar levels is to eat more refined carbohydrates.

Even a few hours a day of sleep deprivation for a week can significantly increase cortisol and insulin. Can the Zone Diet overcome these negative hormonal consequences? To test this hypothesis, I did a small clinical study with medical interns who were ready to begin a two-week period of continuous sleep deprivation in hospital wards. During this time of high stress, they would have only about four hours of total sleep per night. The interns were split into two groups. One group ate at the hospital cafeteria, and the other group received prepared Zone meals and were given 2.5 grams of EPA and DHA every day. After two weeks, those interns eating at the hospital cafeteria were gaining waist circumference, and their cholesterol and triglyceride levels were increasing. The interns getting the Zone meals and fish oil were actually losing weight and seeing improved blood lipid levels.

However, the most interesting outcome was the mental cognition of the interns. After two weeks of sleep deprivation, those eating at the hospital cafeteria were operating at a cognitive level of a typical eighty-five-year-old, based on a standardized word recall test. Those eating the Zone meals and taking the fish oil were operating at the same mental cognition level as they were before the two weeks of constant sleep deprivation.

Although sleep deprivation is here to stay, your diet can greatly reduce the adverse hormonal consequences that come with it.

Improved Temperature Control

Another unintended consequence of our advancing technology is our growing demand for increased temperature comfort. There is an ambient temperature thermoneutral zone (TNZ) in which energy expenditure is minimized to maintain your internal temperature. If the ambient temperature is below the TNZ, you expend energy by shivering to try to maintain your core temperature. If the ambient temperature is above the TNZ, you eat less food. With the advent of improved heating during the winter and air-conditioning in the summer, we can now keep ourselves in the TNZ year round. The end result is that we tend to eat more and expend less energy to stay comfortable. It's routinely done in livestock management to maximize weight gain, and it apparently is having similar effects on humans. It's highly unlikely that Americans are going to turn off their air conditioners in the summer or turn back their thermostats in the winter. But the one thing we can do is increase satiety so we have less desire to eat once we are in the thermoneutral zone.

Chemical Toxins

Many fat-soluble chemical toxins are also hormonal disruptors. Because these toxins will accumulate in the adipose tissue, their potential to disrupt hormonal signaling is greater in the fat cells than any other cell in the body. In particular, bisphenol A (found in plastic bottles), tributyltin (used as an anti-fouling paint on ships), and PCBs appear to be the worst offenders. These fat-soluble toxins that are concentrated in your fat cells increase the efficiency of the fat trap in genetically susceptible individuals.

Willpower Versus Biology

Our debate about obesity has been increasingly shifting its focus on psychology as opposed to biology. In this view, obesity is simply due to the lack of willpower to restrain oneself from eating too much or not exercising enough.

On the other hand, I focus on the biological factors that have changed in the past twenty-five years, and now virtually guarantee that genetically predisposed individuals will be both hungrier and fatter. The people who are getting much fatter today are the ones who were already overweight to begin with. The ability to accumulate excess fat is just as genetically determined as your ultimate height is. If you are genetically predisposed to accumulate excess fat (you have a fat trap) and are following a pro-inflammatory diet, you will begin uncoupling the balance between hunger and satiety as well as increasing the efficiency of your fat trap, which leads to further weight gain.

The impact of the Perfect Nutritional Storm on increased levels of toxic fat has also resulted in the twin adverse effects of (1) increased levels of endocannabinoids in the brain that tell you to keep eating and (2) increased levels of insulin making the fat trap of those genetically predisposed individuals even more efficient. Our obesity epidemic is due not to lack of willpower but to hormonal changes in those who are genetically susceptible. Now their genes are interacting adversely with their diet. This has nothing to do with willpower. It's just bad luck that can potentially shorten their lives.

Biological Factors that Cause Weight Regain

Losing weight is relatively simple; keeping it off is the difficult part. We are just now learning the biological factors that make weight maintenance so difficult. One is the hormone leptin. This hormone is secreted by the adipose tissue to signal to the brain that fat stores are sufficient and to stop eating.

Soon after leptin was discovered, it was found that injecting this hormone into genetically bred obese mice would reverse their obesity. Perhaps obese people were simply deficient in this hormone and increasing its levels by daily injections would solve their eating problems. Unfortunately, it turns out that obese individuals have leptin resistance, not a leptin deficiency. If the transport of leptin into their brain is compromised, then leptin simply piles up in the bloodstream, never reaching the brain in sufficient levels to signal satiety.

Just as constant exposure to insulin leads to desensitization of insulin receptors, thus increasing insulin resistance, constant exposure to leptin can likewise increase leptin resistance. The fatter you are, the more leptin your brain will be exposed to over a lifetime, and the receptors will become more desensitized to its signal. Another cause of this leptin resistance is an increase in C-reactive protein (CRP), due to increased silent inflammation. CRP binds to leptin and prevents its entry into the brain. Another factor is an increase in triglyceride levels that also reduce leptin's entry into the brain. Reduce silent inflammation, and you reduce both CRP levels and triglyceride levels. The end result is greater satiety as more leptin reaches its receptors in the brain.

Unfortunately, studies have shown that when obese individuals lose weight, their problems with leptin sensitivity often remain. With the loss of body fat, leptin levels drop, but the brain perceives this as a leptin deficiency and sends out hormonal signals to consume more food to build up fat stores. It also turns out that during weight loss, their cells become more efficient in making adenosine triphosphate (ATP), so fewer incoming calories are needed to maintain cellular function. This leads to a twofold whammy: the brain is telling you to eat more as it perceives a leptin deficiency, yet fewer calories are needed to make the chemical energy (ATP) the body requires. The excess calories not needed for ATP production are now converted into fat that can be accumulated in the fat trap. This is another reason weight maintenance is so difficult—unless other hormonal factors that lead to satiety can be activated.

I feel the real cause of our increased hunger is the increased levels of toxic fat (AA), especially in the brain. Arachidonic acid (AA) is the building block for the group of eicosanoids known as endocannabinoids. These are the hormones that bind to receptors in the brain that produce increased hunger (that is, the munchies). An experimental drug (Rimonabant) inhibits the binding of endocannabinoids to their receptors and as a result causes weight loss. Unfortunately, the same drug has a few side effects, such as suicidal thoughts, anxiety, and depression, that have prevented its approval in the United States.

This is why high-dose fish oil rich in EPA can play a significant role in satiety. As the EPA enters the brain, it can inhibit the binding of these endocannabinoids to their receptors in the brain because of its close structural similarity to AA. However, EPA exists in the brain only for a short period of time (about four to six hours) before it is converted into DHA (this is why you find little EPA in the brain). But during this time it is a powerful suppressor of hunger. Taking high-dose fish oil after a meal is an effective way to quell hunger for the next four to six hours. This was one of the secrets for Manuel Uribe's great weight-loss success; he was taking high-dose fish oil (providing about 5 grams of EPA) after every meal. The end result was that he was never hungry. For most people, their real hunger comes about two hours after dinner. If you take about 5 grams of EPA right after dinner, then these munchies as you watch TV will virtually disappear.

Weight Loss Versus Weight Maintenance

There is a very big difference between losing weight and keeping it off. Some people have lost hundreds of pounds only to gain them back. In an effort to try to find what the factors that allow successful long-term weight maintenance are, the National Weight Control Registry (NWCR) was established in 1994. The NWCR is open to people who have lost thirty pounds and have kept it off for more than a year. Although it only has about six thousand registered members, the NWCR provides very useful information about those who have successful weight-maintenance strategies. Keep in mind that the average person in the NWCR is still overweight (average BMI of about 25) but at least no longer obese (the average starting BMI was about 35). Those who are the most successful (losing more than sixty pounds and keeping it off for more than five years) report eating less than 1,400 calories a day in addition to exercising an hour a day to burn off another 400 calories. This means they have to net less than 1,000 calories per day just to stay overweight. These people have a genetic predisposition for weight gain that they have to fight for a lifetime. They are maintaining their weight by depleting their ATP levels by calorie restriction and increased exercise. It's a dangerous game to play because any additional

ATP they need has to come from cannibalism of their muscles and organs. Again, it's not fair, but it's in their genes.

To Lose Weight, Simply Exercise More

It is very easy to choose lack of exercise as the villain of the obesity epidemic since you don't have to tell anyone to stop doing anything; you only have to add something to your lifestyle. This approach, in theory, allows you to eat whatever you want if you exercise enough. In essence, it is the real basis of the new USDA Food Pyramid, which can be summarized as "eat *more* and exercise more." Unfortunately, you come up against the 80/20 rule for weight loss: 80 percent of your weight-loss success will come from your diet and the other 20 percent from exercise. Here are some of the realities of calorie consumption. About 70 percent of your daily calorie needs are required for your resting metabolic rate (RMR)—providing enough chemical energy (ATP) just to run your body. Another 10 percent of your daily calories are used to digest food and convert those calories to ATP to run the body. This leaves about 20 percent of your daily calories for moving your body around. This is where I get the 80/20 rule.

If you start exercising more, then you need to produce more ATP. If you can't effectively access this extra ATP from your stored fat, then you have to either eat more calories or begin cannibalizing your muscles and organs to get needed energy for the body's extra demand for more ATP for your increased exercise. If you decide at the same time to eat fewer calories, then your only option is cannibalization.

This is why reducing incoming calories is always more successful in promoting weight loss than increasing daily exercise. However, that is only true if you aren't hungry between meals. This means whatever diet you choose to follow has to (1) reduce endocannabinoids, (2) reduce insulin levels, and (3) increase satiety at the same time. A pretty tall task. This is why people in published long-term clinical studies initially lose weight by eating less and exercising more. Remember, the people who enter these studies are highly motivated to succeed, meaning they have lots of willpower. However, increased exercise requires more ATP. So where does the extra ATP come from if you have not reduced the efficiency of your fat trap? The answer is cannibalization of your muscles and organs. Eventually you reach an impossible situation where significant organ damage is beginning to occur, and the only intelligent response is to start eating more (as well as exercising less) to maintain sufficient levels of ATP to stop further cannibalization. The result is that the subjects in these long-term studies generally regain the weight. This puts them back into an energy balance where incoming calories that can be easily converted into ATP balances the ATP required to survive and move around.

This was also true of the two large-scale children studies (described in chapter 4), in which the intervention group exercised more that the control group. After several years, the children who exercised more were exactly the same weight as those who didn't exercise nearly as much.

Don't get me wrong. There are many good reasons to exercise: it improves cardiovascular endurance; reduces the lipotoxicity associated with diabetes and heart disease, thus allowing for longer life; can provide social involvement; and improves mood. But weight loss is not one of those good reasons. Frankly, it is much easier to lose weight by reducing your caloric intake by 500 calories a day, following the Zone Diet, than by burning 500 calories a day on a treadmill, which increases appetite.

Taking weight off is relatively easy, but keeping weight off is going to be a lifetime challenge, especially if you are genetically predisposed to store dietary calories as extra fat. However, the real goal is not weight loss but keeping silent inflammation under control if you want to live a longer and better life. This can be achieved only by following an anti-inflammatory diet that is keeping the production of toxic fat to a minimum level.

Putting all of these biological factors together, you begin to see why most people fail to maintain initial weight loss. All of these biological factors can be modified to your benefit by reducing silent inflammation using the combination of the Zone Diet and high-dose fish oil, thus tilting the balance of satiety and hunger back in your favor. Only then can long-term weight maintenance become a reality.

Summary

Even with the right dietary tools, it's going to be difficult to win your lifelong struggle against toxic fat. If you want to go back to living a 1920s lifestyle (no vegetable oils, few refined carbohydrates, no TV, no Internet, no fat-soluble toxins, no air-conditioning, little heat, and plenty of sleep), then silent inflammation and its most obvious fellow travelers of obesity, type 2 diabetes, and heart disease would virtually disappear. Of course, few of us are going to want to live that way today. However, understanding the nature of obstacles presented by modern life and dietary ways to circumvent them gives you a leg up in the lifelong struggle to keep silent inflammation under control.

CHAPTER 12

The Coming Reckoning

IN LESS THAN A DECADE, IT IS VERY POSSIBLE THAT AMERICA WILL be close to bankruptcy caused by raging inflation coupled with economic stagnation caused by the breakdown of our health-care system.

The time of reckoning will begin in 2011, and the economic consequences for the entire country will be in full force by 2016. What's so special about the year 2011? That is the year when the first of the baby boomers can begin accessing the virtually free health-care benefits of Medicare, including the newest and most expensive drugs.

It was easy for politicians to promise all of these wondrous medical benefits to younger voters in the twentieth century because they would not be in office when the time came to pay for them. But starting in 2011, the payment comes due. Today the unfunded liabilities of Medicare are greater than $30 trillion. That number is so staggering that no one wants to talk about it. To put that $30 trillion into perspective, it is equivalent to rebuilding New Orleans one-hundred-fifty times or fighting thirty Iraqi wars.

When the first tidal wave of aging baby boomers hits the Medicare rolls in 2011, the medical bills will start to pile up quickly because they are a lot sicker than we ever thought. The politicians will have several options when this happens. One option is that the newly eligible Medicare recipients could be asked to wait a few more years before getting their free medical care. Another option is asking the younger working generation to accept a massive increase in their Medicare taxes to pay for the newly arriving costs to the virtually nonexistent Medicare trust fund. Neither of these options will be likely because these people vote. The last option is the one that most politicians tend to fall back on in difficult fiscal times—print more money.

There is even more trouble coming right behind the rapid rise of the Medicare costs. This is the current health of our children. It has been estimated that one of every three children born after the year 2000 will develop type 2 diabetes. This is the most expensive chronic disease to treat, and once you develop type 2 diabetes, this disease takes ten to fifteen years off your potential life expectancy. This may be the first time in American history that parents will start outliving their children.

Virtually every obese pediatric child whom I have tested has had high AA/EPA ratios in their blood. This is the definition of Toxic Fat Syndrome. This means only one thing: chronic disease (such as type 2 diabetes) will be occurring at earlier and earlier ages in these children. We are already seeing a rapid rise of childhood neurological disorders such as depression and attention deficit disorder, as well as asthma and allergies. Our children are like canaries in the coal mine. Their worsening health is indicative that the epidemic of Toxic Fat Syndrome is going to rob Americans of their wellness at a much earlier age in life.

These medical problems are not confined to the United States; they are becoming a worldwide phenomenon. At the World Diabetes Congress in South Africa in December 2006, it was projected that the worldwide incidence of type 2 diabetes will rise to 380 million people by 2025. The current total of worldwide diabetic populations stands at 246 million, and it was only 30 million twenty years ago. More than 80 percent of the projected 2025 total of diabetics will be in poor- and middle-income countries that simply don't have the wealth to pay for the massive costs that come with diabetes.

In the United States each diabetic patient costs more than $10,000 per year to treat. This is why nearly 50 percent of the worldwide treatment costs of diabetes are expended in the United States, although we have only 8 percent of the world's diabetic population. Currently about 20 million people in the United States have diabetes, but that number is dwarfed by the more than 80 million diabetics in India and China. The World Health Organization states that diabetes, and the associated heart disease and strokes that come with it, will be a major drag on world economic growth.

It is estimated that by 2025 China will lose $500 billion annually in national income, and Russia will lose nearly $300 billion per year due to treating diabetes-related diseases. These are costs that neither country is prepared to pay. It is not clear whether even America can pay the costs that come with our own ever-increasing diabetes epidemic caused by Toxic Fat Syndrome. Even more striking is the fact that the annual worldwide death toll related to diabetes is now estimated at 3.8 million people. This is more than the worldwide death toll of HIV and malaria combined. As Martin Silink, the president of the International Diabetes Federation, has stated, "This is an epidemic that seems to have crept up on people. The enormity of the epidemic has suddenly become apparent." Well, it didn't exactly creep up because type 2 diabetes is preceded by at least a decade of the presence of Toxic Fat Syndrome.

As I have tried to put forward in this book, the underlying cause of these growing health ills on a worldwide stage is the growing epidemic of Toxic Fat Syndrome. It doesn't come from sloth or gluttony (actually these are consequences of the increased efficiency of the fat trap), but it is caused by rapid changes in our current pro-inflammatory diet that are now interacting adversely with our genes. The end result is silent inflammation that can spread like a cancer to every organ in your body. As it does, chronic disease begins to appear at earlier and earlier ages.

Yet all of these dire scenarios can be reversed rapidly, not by any drug, but simply by your diet. In fact, there is no known drug that can reverse silent inflammation caused by increasing levels of toxic fat in our bodies (although several can accelerate it).

I have outlined in this book, and in many of the other books that I have written, the relative ease of the dietary changes needed to reverse silent inflammation. These are not temporary changes; you have to incorporate them for a lifetime. Remember, that is the real meaning of *diet*, which comes from the Greek root that means "way of life." That truly describes the Zone Diet. It is a way of life to control silent inflammation, and that has to be a lifelong commitment.

There are many formidable obstacles in your struggle to control silent inflammation, but once you know what they are, you can address them. Some are obvious; others are subtle. Some are imbedded in your genes. It means that reversing Toxic Fat Syndrome throughout your body is going to be a lifelong process.

As difficult as the obstacles may be, I remain optimistic that we can turn back the epidemic of Toxic Fat Syndrome because it is ultimately an individual struggle that can begin one person at a time. This is how all revolutions are started. The end result is a longer and better life, which is well worth the effort.

CHAPTER 13

Anti-Inflammatory Meals to Reverse Toxic Fat Syndrome in Less Than 30 Days

OXIC FAT SYNDROME IS ULTIMATELY CAUSED BY YOUR DIET, WHICH means it can be reversed by your diet, but only if that diet is an anti-inflammatory one like the Zone Diet.

What I have provided here is a 28-day program to begin to reverse Toxic Fat Syndrome for both men and women. These meals were developed using the Zone Food Block Method described in chapter 10 and in greater detail in appendix H.

The recipes come from my various books and from individuals who have submitted recipes to my Web sites. Hundreds of other Zone meals can be found in *Zone Meals in Seconds, The Soy Zone, Mastering the Zone, Zone Meals in Minutes,* and *The Top 100 Zone Foods.* Even more recipes can be found on my Web site, Zonediet.com.

Each recipe is a 3-block meal for a typical woman. Also given is what is needed to convert the recipe to a 4-block meal for the typical man.

Here are a few helpful hints to get you started:

1. Each recipe calls for a different type of fruit. Feel free to use one or two fruits throughout the week if you find it more economical and convenient.

2. Also feel free to use precooked chicken, such as Perdue Short Cuts, for certain recipes.

3. Cook more than one portion at a time if you feel so inclined. Recipes, such as Zone Chili or Meatloaf, can be doubled or tripled. You might want to cook twice as much chicken breast as you need. Use the first portion for the recipe you are following and the rest for a recipe that also calls for cooked chicken, such as chicken salad.

4. Use frozen pre-chopped vegetables, such as onions, peppers, and broccoli florets. When a recipe calls for a little bit of this and a little bit of that, you can just pull the correct portion out of the freezer.

5. If chopping vegetables is still too time-consuming, consider the favorable carbohydrates that give you the most cluck for the buck. For example, ¼ cup hummus, ½ cup tomato sauce, ¼ cup cooked lentils, and ¼ cup of garbanzo, black, or kidney beans each equals one block.

6. I will feature a limited amount of unfavorable carbohydrates in the first week of the program as you wean yourself off bread and other high glycemic-load carbohydrates.

7. Feel free to take the recipes out of sequence until you find a plan that suits you.

8. Finally, take adequate levels of EPA (eicosapentaenoic acid) and DHA (docosahexaenoic acid) on a daily basis.

28-Day Toxic Fat Syndrome Reversal Plan

WEEK ONE: Day 1

BREAKFAST
> Scrambled Eggs and Bacon

Ingredients for women

1 ounce Canadian bacon or
    3 turkey bacon strips
Vegetable spray
4 egg whites or 1/2 cup egg substitute
2/3 teaspoon olive oil
1 teaspoon milk, optional

Optional spices

1/8 teaspoon dill
1/8 teaspoon chives
1/8 teaspoon hot sauce
Salt and pepper to taste
Sprinkling of low-fat mozzarella cheese
1 cup grapes
1/2 slice rye toast
1 teaspoon old-fashioned
    peanut butter

Ingredients for men

1 ounce Canadian bacon or
    3 turkey bacon strips
Vegetable spray
6 egg whites or 3/4 cup egg substitute
1 teaspoon olive oil
1 teaspoon milk, optional

Optional spices

1/8 teaspoon dill
1/8 teaspoon chives
1/8 teaspoon hot sauce
Salt and pepper to taste
Sprinkling of low-fat mozzarella cheese
11/2 cups grapes
1/2 slice rye toast
1 teaspoon old-fashioned
    peanut butter

Cook the bacon in a skillet over medium heat. Spray a nonstick pan with vegetable spray. While the bacon is cooking, prepare the eggs. Beat the eggs with olive oil, a little milk if desired, and the spices. Scramble the eggs in the prepared pan over medium heat until almost done, and then fold in the cheese. Have grapes and a half slice of toast with peanut butter on the side.

LUNCH
> Seafood Salad

Ingredients for women	*Ingredients for men*
4$^1/_2$ ounces canned seafood	6 ounces canned seafood
(shrimp, crabmeat, or lobster)	(shrimp, crabmeat, or lobster)
1 tablespoon light mayonnaise	4 teaspoons light mayonnaise
$^1/_8$ teaspoon dill	$^1/_8$ teaspoon dill
$^1/_8$ teaspoon garlic powder	$^1/_8$ teaspoon garlic powder
Salt and pepper to taste	Salt and pepper to taste
1 mini pita pocket, cut off top edge	1 mini pita pocket, cut off top edge
1 cup frozen raspberries, thawed	2 cups frozen raspberries, thawed

Mix the seafood with mayonnaise and spices. Stuff into the mini pocket. Have the raspberries on the side.

Late-Afternoon Zone Snack

(Potential Zone snacks for this 28-day plan are listed at the end of this chapter, beginning on page 229.)

DINNER
> Chili

Ingredients for women	*Ingredients for men*
4$^1/_2$ ounces lean ground meat	6 ounces lean ground meat
(beef or turkey)	(beef or turkey)
1 teaspoon olive oil	1$^1/_3$ teaspoons olive oil
$^1/_4$ cup minced onions	$^1/_4$ cup minced onions
$^1/_4$ cup chopped mushrooms	$^1/_4$ cup chopped mushrooms
$^1/_4$ cup chopped green bell pepper	$^1/_4$ cup chopped green bell pepper

Chili powder, oregano, and pepper to taste	Chili powder, oregano, and pepper to taste
1/4 cup kidney beans, drained and rinsed	1/2 cup kidney beans, drained and rinsed
1 cup canned crushed tomatoes with liquid	1 cup canned crushed tomatoes with liquid
Sprinkling of low-fat Monterey Jack cheese	Sprinkling of low-fat Monterey Jack cheese
1 peach	1 peach

In a nonstick pan, brown meat in oil over medium heat. Add minced onions, mushrooms, bell peppers, and spices. Cook for fifteen minutes or until vegetables are soft, stirring often. Add the kidney beans and tomatoes. Cook for ten to fourteen minutes. Sprinkle with cheese before serving. Have peach on the side.

Late-Evening Zone Snack

(Potential Zone snacks for this 28-day plan are listed at the end of this chapter, beginning on page 229.)

Fish Oil Requirements: Take at least 2.5 grams of EPA and DHA sometime during the day. Take more according to the guidelines in chapter 9 if you have the complications associated with Toxic Fat Syndrome.

Day 2

BREAKFAST
❯ Old-Fashioned Oatmeal

Ingredients for women	*Ingredients for men*
1 cup cooked steel-cut oatmeal	1 1/3 cups cooked steel-cut oatmeal

Nutmeg	Nutmeg
Cinnamon	Cinnamon
$1/3$ ounce protein powder (7 grams)	$2/3$ ounce protein powder (14 grams)
1 tablespoon slivered almonds	4 teaspoons slivered almonds
2 ounces Canadian bacon or six turkey bacon strips	2 ounces Canadian bacon or six turkey bacon strips

Cook oatmeal according to package instructions, adding nutmeg and cinnamon to taste. Stir in protein powder and almonds. Prepare bacon and serve on the side.

LUNCH
> Cheeseburger

Ingredients for women	*Ingredients for men*
Vegetable spray	Vegetable spray
$4^1/2$ ounces lean ground beef or turkey	6 ounces lean ground beef or turkey
Salt, pepper, and spices of your choice to taste	Salt, pepper, and spices of your choice to taste
1 slice reduced-fat cheese	1 slice reduced-fat cheese
1 teaspoon reduced-fat mayonnaise	2 teaspoons reduced-fat mayonnaise
$1/2$ piece rye bread	1 piece rye bread
Tomato slice, lettuce leaf, onion slice, optional	Tomato slice, lettuce leaf, onion slice, optional
1 apple	1 apple
12 peanuts	12 peanuts

Spray a nonstick pan with vegetable spray. Combine the ground beef or turkey with the seasonings and form a patty. Cook the patty in the prepared pan over medium heat, about five minutes per side. Top with cheese and let it melt a bit if desired. Spread mayonnaise on bread and top with hamburger, tomato, lettuce, and onion slice. Have apple and peanuts on the side.

Late-Afternoon Zone Snack

DINNER
> BBQ chicken

Ingredients for women	Ingredients for men
3 ounces boneless, skinless chicken breast	4 ounces boneless, skinless chicken breast
2 lemon slices	2 lemon slices
2 onion slices	2 onion slices
1 to 2 teaspoons barbecue sauce	1 to 2 teaspoons barbecue sauce
Spinach	Spinach
$1/2$ cup sliced celery	$1/2$ cup sliced celery
1 cup sliced cucumber	1 cup sliced cucumber
$3/4$ cup sliced onions (or any combination of vegetables, adding up to one block as outlined in appendix H)	$3/4$ cup sliced onions (or any combination of vegetables, adding up to one block as outlined in appendix H)
1 teaspoon olive oil	$1^1/3$ teaspoons olive oil
Vinegar to taste	Vinegar to taste
$1^1/2$ cups cooked green beans	$1^1/2$ cups cooked green beans
1 cup strawberries	1 cup blueberries

Preheat oven to 450 degrees. Cover chicken breast with lemon and onion slices. Bake for fifteen minutes. Reduce heat to 350 degrees. Baste with barbecue sauce. Cook for ten to fifteen minutes or until done. While cooking, toss the spinach, celery, cucumber, and onions in a bowl. Sprinkle with olive oil and vinegar. Have the chicken with beans, fruit, and salad on the side.

Late-Evening Zone Snack

Fish Oil Requirements: Take at least 2.5 grams of EPA and DHA sometime during the day. Take more according to the guidelines in chapter 9 if you have the complications associated with Toxic Fat Syndrome.

Day 3

BREAKFAST
> Fruit Salad

Ingredients for women	*Ingredients for men*
3/4 cup low-fat cottage cheese	1 cup low-fat cottage cheese
1 cup strawberries	1 cup strawberries
1/2 cup grapes	1 cup grapes
1/3 cup unsweetened mandarin oranges	1/3 cup unsweetened mandarin oranges
3 macadamia nuts, crushed	4 macadamia nuts, crushed

Combine the ingredients in a large bowl and enjoy.

LUNCH
> Chef Salad

Ingredients for women	*Ingredients for men*
Bed of lettuce	Bed of lettuce
1 green bell pepper, sliced	1 green bell pepper, sliced

1 sliced tomato

1/3 cup water chestnuts

1/4 cup chickpeas

(or any combination of vegetables, adding up to three blocks as outlined in appendix H)

1 1/2 ounces deli-style turkey breast

1 1/2 ounces deli-style ham

1 ounce low-fat cheese

1 teaspoon olive oil

Vinegar to taste

1 sliced tomato

1/3 cup water chestnuts

1/4 cup chickpeas

(or any combination of vegetables, adding up to three blocks as outlined in appendix H)

3 ounces deli-style turkey breast

1 1/2 ounces deli-style ham

1 ounce low-fat cheese

1 1/3 teaspoons olive oil

Vinegar to taste

1 plum (for dessert)

Combine the lettuce, bell pepper, tomatoes, chestnuts, and chickpeas in a large bowl. Top with turkey, ham, and cheese. Combine oil and vinegar and whisk well. Pour dressing over salad and toss.

Late-Afternoon Zone Snack

DINNER

> Foiled Fish

Ingredients for women

Vegetable spray

4 1/2 ounces flounder fillet (or your choice)

2 tablespoons Parmesan cheese

Freshly ground pepper to taste

Dash of lemon juice

Chopped onion, to taste

Ingredients for men

Vegetable spray

6 ounces flounder fillet (or your choice)

2 tablespoons Parmesan cheese

Freshly ground pepper to taste

Dash of lemon juice

Chopped onion, to taste

2 cups cooked asparagus	2 cups cooked asparagus
1 tablespoon slivered almonds	4 teaspoons slivered almonds
1 cup raspberries	2 cups raspberries

Lightly spray the center of a large piece of aluminum foil with vegetable spray. Put fish in the center of the foil. Top with cheese, pepper, lemon juice, and onion. Fold foil over fish, leaving space around the fish. Carefully turn up and seal the ends and the middle so that the juices don't leak out. Bake at 425 degrees for eighteen minutes. When done, carefully open foil to prevent steam burns. Have asparagus topped with almonds and raspberries on the side.

Late-Evening Zone Snack

Fish Oil Requirements: Take at least 2.5 grams of EPA and DHA sometime during the day. Take more according to the guidelines in chapter 9 if you have the complications associated with Toxic Fat Syndrome.

Day 4

BREAKFAST
> Feta omelet

Ingredients for women	Ingredients for men
Vegetable spray	Vegetable spray
4 egg whites or $1/2$ cup egg substitute (Add a bit of milk if desired)	6 egg whites or $3/4$ cup egg substitute (Add a bit of milk if desired)
1 ounce low-fat feta cheese, crumbled	1 ounce low-fat feta cheese, crumbled
9 sliced olives	12 sliced olives
$2/3$ cup cooked steel-cut oatmeal	1 cup cooked steel-cut oatmeal
$1/2$ cup blueberries	$1/2$ cup blueberries

Spray nonstick pan with vegetable spray. Scramble eggs in pan over medium heat and fold in feta cheese and olives. Serve oatmeal on the side, topped with blueberries.

LUNCH
> Chicken Salad Sandwich

Ingredients for women	*Ingredients for men*
3 ounces chicken breast (canned may be used), shredded	4 ounces chicken breast (canned may be used), shredded
1 tablespoon light mayonnaise	4 teaspoons light mayonnaise
Salt and pepper to taste	Salt and pepper to taste
1 stalk celery, chopped	1 stalk celery, chopped
1 cup sliced grapes	1 cup sliced grapes
1 mini pita pocket or $1/2$ slice rye bread	1 mini pita pocket or $1/2$ slice rye bread
Lettuce, tomato slice, optional	Lettuce, tomato slice, optional
	1 tangerine (for dessert)

Mix chicken with mayonnaise, salt and pepper, celery, and grapes. Put in pita pocket and add tomato slice and lettuce.

Late-Afternoon Zone Snack

DINNER
> Meatloaf

Ingredients for women	*Ingredients for men*
$4^1/2$ ounces lean ground beef or ground turkey	6 ounces lean ground beef or ground turkey

2 tablespoons egg substitute	2 tablespoons egg substitute
1 teaspoon breadcrumbs	1 teaspoon breadcrumbs
1 tablespoon catsup	1 tablespoon catsup
$1/3$ cup finely chopped onions	$1/3$ cup finely chopped onions
Dash Worcestershire sauce	Dash Worcestershire sauce
$1/4$ teaspoon thyme	$1/4$ teaspoon thyme
Pepper to taste	Pepper to taste
Bed of lettuce	Bed of lettuce
$1/2$ cup artichoke hearts, in a jar or canned, and	$1/2$ cup artichoke hearts, in a jar or canned, and
2 cups chopped mushrooms or other vegetables, adding up to one block)	2 cups chopped mushrooms or other vegetables, adding up to one block)
1 teaspoon olive oil	$1^{1}/3$ teaspoons olive oil
Vinegar to taste	Vinegar to taste
2 cups chopped cooked zucchini	2 cups chopped cooked zucchini
$1/2$ apple	1 apple

Combine ground meat, egg substitute, breadcrumbs, catsup, onions, Worcestershire sauce, thyme, and pepper in large bowl and mix well. Form into a shallow loaf and place in microwave-safe dish. Cover with waxed paper. Microwave on medium for ten to fifteen minutes or until done, or bake in 350-degree oven until cooked throughout. While cooking, combine lettuce, artichoke hearts, and mushrooms in a large bowl. In a small bowl, combine oil and vinegar and whisk well. Pour the dressing over the salad and toss. Serve salad, zucchini, and apple on the side.

Late-Evening Zone Snack

Fish Oil Requirements: Take at least 2.5 grams of EPA and DHA sometime during the day. Take more according to the guidelines in chapter 9 if you have the complications associated with Toxic Fat Syndrome.

DAY 5

BREAKFAST

> Skillet Breakfast Hash

Ingredients for women	Ingredients for men
Chopped onion to taste	Chopped onion to taste
Chopped green bell pepper to taste	Chopped green bell pepper to taste
Chopped mushrooms to taste	Chopped mushrooms to taste
1 teaspoon olive oil	$1^1/_3$ teaspoons olive oil
3 ounces cooked meat	4 ounces cooked meat
(roast beef, chicken, ham; canned is fine)	(roast beef, chicken, ham; canned is fine)
$^1/_3$ cup diced cooked potato	$^1/_3$ cup diced cooked potato
$1^1/_2$ cups chopped tomato	$1^1/_2$ cups chopped tomato
Salt and pepper to taste	Salt and pepper to taste
Worcestershire sauce to taste	Worcestershire sauce to taste
$^1/_2$ grapefruit	$^1/_2$ grapefruit
	$^3/_4$ cup V8 juice

In a nonstick pan, sauté onion, bell pepper, and mushrooms over medium heat until tender. Add meat, potato, tomato, salt and pepper, and Worcestershire sauce. Cook, stirring often until heated through. Have grapefruit on the side. (If you want to eliminate the potato, increase to 1 grapefruit.)

LUNCH
> Open-Faced BLT Sandwich

Ingredients for women	Ingredients for men
Vegetable spray	Vegetable spray
2 ounces lean Canadian bacon or 6 turkey bacon strips	2 ounces lean Canadian bacon or 6 turkey bacon strips
2 teaspoons low-fat mayonnaise	1 tablespoon low-fat mayonnaise
1 piece rye bread	1 piece rye bread
1 ounce low-fat cheese	2 ounces low-fat cheese
Lettuce	Lettuce
1 tomato slice	1 tomato slice
$1/2$ orange	1 orange
6 peanuts	6 peanuts

Spray a nonstick pan with vegetable spray. Cook bacon over medium heat. Spread mayonnaise on the bread. Add cheese, lettuce, and tomato. Have orange and peanuts on the side.

Late-Afternoon Zone Snack

DINNER
> Turkey Scaloppini with Mushrooms

Ingredients for women	Ingredients for men
1 teaspoon olive oil, divided	$1^{1}/_{3}$ teaspoons olive oil, divided
3 ounces turkey breast, sliced in strips	4 ounces turkey breast, sliced in strips
$3/4$ cup finely chopped onion	$3/4$ cup finely chopped onion

2 teaspoons cider vinegar
$1/8$ teaspoon lemon herb seasoning
2 cups thinly sliced mushrooms
$2/3$ cup unsweetened applesauce
2 teaspoons cornstarch
1 teaspoon orange extract
$1/8$ teaspoon dill
$1/4$ teaspoon cinnamon
1 cup lemon- or lime-flavored
   water

2 teaspoons cider vinegar
$1/8$ teaspoon lemon herb seasoning
2 cups thinly sliced mushrooms
$2/3$ cup unsweetened applesauce
2 teaspoons cornstarch
1 teaspoon orange extract
$1/8$ teaspoon dill
$1/4$ teaspoon cinnamon
1 cup lemon- or lime-flavored
   water
$1/2$ pear (for dessert)

Add $1/2$ teaspoon oil in nonstick sauté pan over medium heat. Sauté turkey with onion, cider vinegar, and lemon herb seasoning. Sauté until turkey is cooked through. In second sauté pan, heat remaining oil and sauté mushrooms for three to five minutes. Add remaining ingredients and sauté until liquid is thickened. (Mix cornstarch with a little water to dissolve it before adding to saucepan.) Spoon mushroom mixture onto serving plate and top with turkey.

Late-Evening Zone Snack

Fish Oil Requirements: Take at least 2.5 grams of EPA and DHA sometime during the day. Take more according to the guidelines in chapter 9 if you have the complications associated with Toxic Fat Syndrome.

Day 6

BREAKFAST

> Eggs and Muffin

Ingredients for women	Ingredients for men
4 egg whites or $1/2$ cup egg substitute	6 egg whites or $3/4$ cup egg substitute
1 teaspoon olive oil	$1^1/3$ teaspoons olive oil
$1/2$ English muffin	$1/2$ English muffin
1 ounce lean Canadian bacon	1 ounce lean Canadian bacon
$1/2$ orange	1 orange

Beat egg whites and olive oil, adding a little milk if desired. Spray a nonstick pan with vegetable spray, and then scramble eggs over medium heat. Toast English muffin. Follow package instructions to cook Canadian bacon. Place bacon on English muffin and top with eggs. Have orange on the side.

LUNCH

> Grilled Chicken Salad

Ingredients for women	Ingredients for men
Bed of romaine lettuce	Bed of romaine lettuce
2 cups sliced mushrooms	2 cups sliced mushrooms
$1^1/2$ cups sliced tomatoes	$1^1/2$ cups sliced tomatoes
$3/4$ cup chopped onions	$3/4$ cup chopped onions
1 teaspoon olive oil	$1^1/3$ teaspoons olive oil
Vinegar to taste	Vinegar to taste
Lemon juice	Lemon juice
Worcestershire sauce to taste	Worcestershire sauce to taste
Pepper to taste	Pepper to taste

4$\frac{1}{2}$ ounces deli-style chicken	6 ounces deli-style chicken
Grated Parmesan cheese	Grated Parmesan cheese
$\frac{1}{2}$ apple	1 apple

Toss together the lettuce, mushrooms, tomatoes, and onions. In a small bowl, combine the oil and vinegar and whisk to combine. Drizzle salad dressing over the salad. Add lemon juice and season with Worcestershire sauce. Grind pepper over the salad. Add chicken and top with sprinkling of Parmesan cheese. Have apple for dessert.

Late-Afternoon Zone Snack

DINNER
> Pork Medallions with Apple

Ingredients for women	*Ingredients for men*
3 ounces pork medallions or thinly sliced pork chops	4 ounces pork medallions or thinly sliced pork chops
Rosemary to taste	Rosemary to taste
Dijon mustard to coat pork	Dijon mustard to coat pork
$\frac{1}{2}$ apple, sliced	$\frac{1}{2}$ apple, sliced
1 to 2 tablespoons white wine, optional	1 to 2 tablespoons white wine, optional
$\frac{1}{4}$ cup water	$\frac{1}{4}$ cup water
$\frac{1}{2}$ bag mixed salad greens	$\frac{1}{2}$ bag mixed salad greens
2 cups broccoli florets	2 cups broccoli florets
$\frac{1}{4}$ cup chickpeas	$\frac{1}{2}$ cup chickpeas
1 teaspoon olive oil	1$\frac{1}{3}$ teaspoons olive oil
Vinegar to taste	Vinegar to taste
$\frac{1}{4}$ cup grapes	$\frac{1}{4}$ cup grapes

Preheat oven to 450 degrees. Place pork in baking dish in a single layer. Top with rosemary, mustard, and apple slices. Pour wine and water around the pork. Bake for ten minutes. Baste pork with pan juices. Reduce heat to 350 degrees. Continue cooking for ten to fifteen minutes or until pork is white, not pink, inside. Enjoy salad and grapes on the side.

Late-Evening Zone Snack

Fish Oil Requirements: Take at least 2.5 grams of EPA and DHA sometime during the day. Take more according to the guidelines in chapter 9 if you have the complications associated with Toxic Fat Syndrome.

Day 7

BREAKFAST
> Yogurt and Fruit

Ingredients for women	Ingredients for men
1 cup plain low-fat yogurt	1^1/$_2$ cups plain low-fat yogurt
1 cup strawberries	1 cup strawberries
1 tablespoon slivered almonds	4 teaspoons slivered almonds
1 ounce Canadian bacon or 3 turkey bacon strips or 7 grams protein powder stirred into yogurt	1 ounce Canadian bacon or 3 turkey bacon strips or 7 grams protein powder stirred into yogurt

Mix yogurt, strawberries, and almonds. Have bacon on the side.

LUNCH

> Turkey in a Pocket

Ingredients for women	Ingredients for men
1 teaspoon light mayonnaise	1 teaspoon light mayonnaise
1 mini pita pocket	1 mini pita pocket
4$^1/_2$ ounces deli turkey or 3 ounces cooked turkey breast	6 ounces deli turkey or 3 ounces cooked turkey breast
Chopped green bell pepper to taste	Chopped green bell pepper to taste
Chopped tomato to taste	Chopped tomato to taste
6 olives, chopped	9 olives, chopped
1 apple	1$^1/_2$ apples

Spread mayonnaise in the pita pocket. Stuff with turkey, bell pepper, tomatoes, and olives. Have apple on the side.

Late-Afternoon Zone Snack

DINNER

> Vegetarian Stir-Fry

Ingredients for women	Ingredients for men
1 cup vegetable protein crumbles or 4 ounces firm tofu	1$^1/_2$ cups vegetable protein crumbles or 6 ounces firm tofu
1 teaspoon olive oil	1$^1/_3$ teaspoons olive oil
1$^1/_2$ cups chopped onions	1$^1/_2$ cups chopped onions
2 cups broccoli florets	2 cups broccoli florets
2 cups sliced mushrooms	2 cups sliced mushrooms
1 ounce reduced-fat shredded cheese	1 ounce reduced-fat shredded cheese
$^1/_2$ apple	1 apple

If tofu is used, drain and crumble. Sauté tofu or crumbles in olive oil in a nonstick pan over medium heat. Add onions, broccoli, and mushrooms. Stir-fry on medium heat until vegetables are tender. Stir in cheese and heat until the cheese is melted. Have apple for dessert.

Late-Evening Zone Snack

Fish Oil Requirements: Take at least 2.5 grams of EPA and DHA sometime during the day. Take more according to the guidelines in chapter 9 if you have the complications associated with Toxic Fat Syndrome.

WEEK 2: Day 1

BREAKFAST
> Blueberry Ricotta Oatmeal

Ingredients for women	*Ingredients for men*
2/3 cup slow-cooked oatmeal, cooked	1 cup slow-cooked oatmeal, cooked
1/2 cup blueberries	1/2 cup blueberries
3 ounces skim ricotta cheese	4 ounces skim ricotta cheese
3 macadamia nuts, crushed	4 macadamia nuts, crushed

Combine the cooked oatmeal, blueberries, ricotta cheese, and macadamia nuts.

LUNCH
> Chinese Chicken

Ingredients for women	*Ingredients for men*
1/3 cup canned mandarin oranges in water, drained	2/3 cup canned mandarin oranges in water, drained

2 cups lettuce	2 cups lettuce
2 cups spinach	2 cups spinach
$1/4$ cup chopped red bell pepper	$1/4$ cup chopped red bell pepper
$1/4$ cup chopped mushrooms	$1/4$ cup chopped mushrooms
$1/4$ cup chopped cucumber	$1/4$ cup chopped cucumber
2 cups cherry tomatoes	2 cups cherry tomatoes
Vegetable spray	Vegetable spray
3 ounces stir-fried chicken breast, cubed	4 ounces stir-fried chicken breast, cubed
Onion salt to taste	Onion salt to taste
Garlic salt to taste	Garlic salt to taste
Pepper to taste	Pepper to taste
Dill to taste	Dill to taste
$1/2$ cup Zoned Chicken Gravy (see below)	$1/2$ cup Zoned Chicken Gravy (see below)
$1/2$ tablespoon tahini	$1/2$ tablespoon tahini
$1/2$ tablespoon avocado	1 tablespoon avocado
$1/2$ teaspoon sesame oil	$1/2$ teaspoon sesame oil
3 peanuts	6 peanuts

Combine mandarin oranges, lettuce, spinach, bell pepper, mushrooms, cucumber, and tomatoes in large bowl. Spray a nonstick pan with cooking spray. Season chicken breast with the onion salt, garlic salt, pepper, and dill, and stir-fry over medium heat. Mix the gravy with the tahini, avacado, sesame oil, and peanuts for dressing. Add chicken to salad. Pour dressing and toss.

> Zoned Chicken Gravy

$2^1/2$ cups strong chicken stock
1 tablespoon white wine, optional
3 cups chopped onions

¹/₂ teaspoon chopped garlic
¹/₂ teaspoon celery salt
1 teaspoon dried parsley flakes
Salt and pepper to taste
8 teaspoons cornstarch

Combine chicken stock, white wine (if using), onions, garlic, celery salt, parsley, and salt and pepper in a small saucepan. Mix cornstarch with a little cold water to dissolve it; then add with other ingredients. Heat sauce mixture to a simmer, transfer to a storage container, let cool, and refrigerate. This sauce may be refrigerated for up to five days, or if you prefer, the sauce may be frozen and thawed for later use. (Although the sauce is freeze-thaw stable, after the sauce has been frozen and thawed, it may need to be stirred to reincorporate the small amount of moisture that forms on the sauce during the freezing and thawing process.)

Note: Each cup of Zoned Chicken Gravy contains one carbohydrate Zone block. There are no protein or fat blocks in this sauce recipe.

Late-Afternoon Zone Snack

DINNER
> Broiled Fish

Ingredients for women	*Ingredients for men*
4¹/₂ ounces fish fillet of your choice	6 ounces fish fillet of your choice
1 teaspoon olive oil	1¹/₃ teaspoons olive oil
Lemon or ginger slices	Lemon or ginger slices
2 tomatoes	2 tomatoes

Parmesan cheese to taste	Parmesan cheese to taste
1 1/2 cups cooked green beans	1 1/2 cups cooked green beans
1/2 cup grapes	1 cup grapes

Brush fish with olive oil. Place lemon slices or ginger on top. Broil ten minutes or until fish flakes. Do not turn. Slice tomatoes in half. Sprinkle with Parmesan cheese and broil until softened. Have grapes for dessert.

Late-Evening Zone Snack

Fish Oil Requirements: Take at least 2.5 grams of EPA and DHA sometime during the day. Take more according to the guidelines in chapter 9 if you have the complications associated with Toxic Fat Syndrome.

DAY 2

BREAKFAST
> Soy Patty and Fruit

Ingredients for women	*Ingredients for men*
2 soy sausage patties	2 soy sausage patties
(about 14 grams of protein)	(about 14 grams of protein)
1 ounce low-fat cheese, sliced	2 ounces low-fat cheese, sliced
Fruit salad:	Fruit salad:
2/3 cup mandarin oranges	2/3 cup mandarin oranges
1/2 cup blueberries	1 cup blueberries
1 tablespoon slivered almonds	4 teaspoons slivered almonds

Cook soy patties according to package directions. Add cheese slices and continue to cook briefly until melted. Combine mandarin oranges and blueberries, and sprinkle almonds on top. Serve sausage with fruit salad.

LUNCH
> Pita Pizza with Salad

Ingredients for women	*Ingredients for men*
Vegetable spray	Vegetable spray
2 ounces lean Canadian bacon or 3 ounces lean ground beef	3 ounces lean Canadian bacon or $4^1/2$ ounces lean ground beef
1 cup chopped green bell pepper, divided	1 cup chopped green bell pepper, divided
$^1/_4$ cup chopped onion	$^1/_4$ cup chopped onion
1 mini pita pocket torn in half, yielding two rounds	1 mini pita pocket torn in half, yielding two rounds
$^1/_4$ cup tomato sauce	$^1/_4$ cup tomato sauce
1 ounce low-fat cheese, grated	1 ounce low-fat cheese, grated
Lettuce	Lettuce
$^3/_4$ cup chopped red bell pepper	$^3/_4$ cup chopped red bell pepper
$^1/_2$ cup chopped tomatoes	$^1/_2$ cup chopped tomatoes
1 teaspoon olive oil	$1^1/_3$ teaspoons olive oil
Vinegar to taste	Vinegar to taste
	$^1/_2$ apple (for dessert)

In a nonstick pan, lightly sprayed with vegetable spray, cook bacon or ground beef. In the same pan, sauté $^1/_4$ cup of the chopped green bell pepper and onion to desired degree of tenderness. Put meat, then tomato sauce, then vegetables on pita rounds. Sprinkle each with cheese. Broil until cheese melts. Combine the lettuce, remaining $^3/_4$ cup green bell pepper, red bell pepper, and tomatoes. Combine the oil and vinegar and whisk together. Pour the dressing over the salad. Serve salad on the side.

Late-Afternoon Zone Snack

DINNER
> Chicken Stir-Fry

Ingredients for women	Ingredients for men
3 ounces skinless, boneless chicken breast, cubed	4 ounces skinless, boneless chicken breast, cubed
$2/3$ teaspoon olive oil	1 teaspoon olive oil
2 cups shredded cabbage	2 cups shredded cabbage
1 green bell pepper, sliced	1 green bell pepper, sliced
$1^1/2$ cups sliced onion	$1^1/2$ cups sliced onion
1 tablespoon teriyaki sauce	1 tablespoon teriyaki sauce
6 peanuts	6 peanuts
1 cup strawberries	2 cups strawberries

Sauté chicken in olive oil in a nonstick pan or wok. Add vegetables and sauté until tender-crisp. Add teriyaki sauce and peanuts for the last minute or two. Have strawberries for dessert.

Late-Evening Zone Snack

Fish Oil Requirements: Take at least 2.5 grams of EPA and DHA sometime during the day. Take more according to the guidelines in chapter 9 if you have the complications associated with Toxic Fat Syndrome.

Day 3

BREAKFAST
> Raspberry Lime Smoothie

Ingredients for women	Ingredients for men
1 cup 1 percent milk	$1^1/2$ cups 1 percent milk

1/2 cup plain low-fat yogurt	3/4 cup plain low-fat yogurt
1 cup raspberries	1 cup raspberries
Juice of 1 lime	Juice of 1 lime
1 tablespoon slivered almonds	4 teaspoons slivered almonds
7 grams protein powder	7 grams protein powder

Place all ingredients except protein powder in blender. Blend until smooth; then stir in protein powder. Serve immediately.

LUNCH
❯ Tuna Salad

Ingredients for women	*Ingredients for men*
3 ounces albacore tuna packed in water	4 ounces albacore tuna packed in water
1 tablespoon light mayonnaise	4 teaspoons light mayonnaise
Chopped celery to taste	Chopped celery to taste
1/4 cup canned chickpeas, drained and rinsed	1/2 cup canned chickpeas, drained and rinsed
Bed of lettuce	Bed of lettuce
1 orange	1 orange

Mix tuna, mayonnaise, and celery. Put tuna mixture and chickpeas on a bed of lettuce. Have orange for dessert.

Late-Afternoon Zone Snack

DINNER

> Broiled Salmon

Ingredients for women	*Ingredients for men*
4^1/$_2$ ounces salmon steak, about 1 inch thick	6 ounces salmon steak, about 1 inch thick
1 teaspoon olive oil	1^1/$_3$ teaspoons olive oil
^{1}/$_2$ teaspoon dried rosemary (or to taste)	^{1}/$_2$ teaspoon dried rosemary (or to taste)
^{1}/$_2$ teaspoon dried tarragon (or to taste)	^{1}/$_2$ teaspoon dried tarragon (or to taste)
^{1}/$_2$ teaspoon dried dill (or to taste)	^{1}/$_2$ teaspoon dried dill (or to taste)
2 cups zucchini, washed, ends removed and sliced into ^{1}/$_4$-inch strips	2 cups zucchini, washed, ends removed and sliced into ^{1}/$_4$-inch strips
Salt and pepper to taste	Salt and pepper to taste
2 kiwis	3 kiwis

Preheat broiler. Brush salmon with olive oil and sprinkle with herbs. On a roasting pan or aluminum foil, broil for four to five minutes per side, depending on thickness, turning once. Meanwhile, steam the zucchini in a large pot fitted with a steaming basket. Bring one inch of water to boil. Add zucchini to the basket and steam until tender-crisp, four to six minutes. Season with salt and pepper. Serve kiwis for dessert.

Late-Evening Zone Snack

Fish Oil Requirements: Take at least 2.5 grams of EPA and DHA sometime during the day. Take more according to the guidelines in chapter 9 if you have the complications associated with Toxic Fat Syndrome.

Day 4

BREAKFAST
> Breakfast from Italy

Ingredients for women	*Ingredients for men*
2 egg whites	4 egg whites
1 teaspoon olive oil	1$^{1}/_{3}$ teaspoons olive oil
Salt and pepper to taste	Salt and pepper to taste
1 ounce prosciutto, sliced into small pieces	1 ounce prosciutto, sliced into small pieces
1 ounce feta cheese, crumbled	1 ounce feta cheese, crumbled
Fruit salad:	Fruit salad:
1 orange, in sections	1 orange, in sections
$^{1}/_{2}$ pear, sliced	1 pear, sliced

Scramble eggs in olive oil with salt and pepper to taste. Add prosciutto and cheese. Have orange and pear on the side.

LUNCH
> Vegetarian Burger

Ingredients for women	*Ingredients for men*
1 soy burger patty (approximately 14 grams of protein)	1$^{1}/_{2}$ soy burger patties (approximately 21 grams of protein)
1 ounce reduced-fat cheese	1 ounce reduced-fat cheese
Lettuce and tomato slice	Lettuce and tomato slice
Dill pickle wedge, optional	Dill pickle wedge, optional
Small side salad:	Small side salad:
2 chopped tomatoes	1 chopped tomato
1 green pepper, cut into strips	1 green pepper, cut into strips

| 1 teaspoon olive oil and vinegar to taste | $1^1/_3$ teaspoons olive oil and vinegar to taste |
| 1 cup unsweetened applesauce, sprinkled with cinnamon | 1 cup unsweetened applesauce, sprinkled with cinnamon |

Spray nonstick pan with vegetable spray. Cook burger, following package instructions. Add the side salad, and have the applesauce for dessert.

Late-Afternoon Zone Snack

DINNER
> Shrimp Scampi

Ingredients for women	*Ingredients for men*
$^3/_4$ cup chopped onion	$^3/_4$ cup chopped onion
1 chopped green pepper	1 chopped green pepper
Garlic to taste	Garlic to taste
1 teaspoon olive oil	$1^1/_3$ teaspoons olive oil
$4^1/_2$ ounces shelled shrimp	6 ounces shelled shrimp
$^1/_4$ cup white wine, optional	$^1/_4$ cup white wine, optional
1-2 teaspoons lemon juice	1-2 teaspoons lemon juice
Lemon wedges	Lemon wedges
1 cup steamed asparagus	1 cup steamed asparagus
Salt and pepper to taste	Salt and pepper to taste
$^1/_2$ pear	1 pear

In a nonstick pan, sauté onion, green pepper, and garlic in olive oil until tender. Add shrimp, white wine, and lemon juice. Cook for five minutes, stirring often, until the shrimp is pink. Garnish with lemon wedges. Have asparagus and pear on the side.

Late-Evening Zone Snack

Fish Oil Requirements: Take at least 2.5 grams of EPA and DHA sometime during the day. Take more according to the guidelines in chapter 9 if you have the complications associated with Toxic Fat Syndrome.

Day 5

BREAKFAST

> Easy Breakfast

Ingredients for women	Ingredients for men
1/3 cup cooked steel-cut oats	2/3 cup cooked steel-cut oats
1/2 cup plain, nonfat yogurt	1/2 cup plain, nonfat yogurt
1/2 cup low-fat cottage cheese	3/4 cup low-fat cottage cheese
Flavoring (lemon, vanilla) to taste	Flavoring (lemon, vanilla) to taste
Spices (cinnamon, allspice, and nutmeg) to taste	Spices (cinnamon, allspice, and nutmeg) to taste
1 packet stevia, optional	1 packet stevia, optional
1/2 cup blueberries or fruit (1 block) of choice	1/2 cup blueberries or fruit (1 block) of choice
1 tablespoon slivered almonds	4 teaspoons slivered almonds

Cook oats according to package directions. Blend together yogurt, cottage cheese, flavoring, spices, and stevia. Layer the oats (press flat), fruit, and yogurt mixture into a serving bowl. Sprinkle with almonds.

LUNCH
> Stuffed Tomato

Ingredients for women

1 tomato

3 ounces albacore tuna packed
    in water

1 tablespoon light mayonnaise

Chopped celery and onion to taste

1 cup mandarin oranges packed
    in water

Ingredients for men

2 tomatoes

4 ounces albacore tuna packed
    in water

4 teaspoons light mayonnaise

Chopped celery and onion to taste

1 cup mandarin oranges packed
    in water

Scoop out tomato. Drain and mix tuna with mayonnaise, celery, and onion. Stuff into tomato. Have fruit for dessert.

Late-Afternoon Zone Snack

DINNER
> Beef Kabobs

Ingredients for women

3 ounces lean beef, cut into cubes

Kabob vegetables, such as onions,
    green peppers, mushrooms, and
    cherry tomatoes

Marinade of your choice

1 spinach salad, consisting of 3
    cups baby spinach, 3/4 cup
    onion, 1 tomato, 2 cups chopped
    mushrooms

Ingredients for men

4 ounces lean beef, cut into cubes

Kabob vegetables, such as onions,
    green peppers, mushrooms, and
    cherry tomatoes

Marinade of your choice

1 spinach salad, consisting of 3
    cups baby spinach, 3/4 cup
    onion, 1 tomato, 2 cups chopped
    mushrooms

1 teaspoon olive oil and vinegar to taste	1 1/3 teaspoons olive oil and vinegar to taste
1 peach	1 apple

Marinate the meat in your favorite marinade or try combining olive oil, low-sodium soy sauce, red wine vinegar, lemon juice, Worcestershire sauce, dry mustard, and pepper. Thread meat and vegetables on skewers. Brush with marinade. Broil three inches from the source of heat (or cook on the barbecue) to your liking. Turn once during cooking time and baste with marinade once or twice. Have salad and fruit on the side.

Late-Evening Zone Snack

Fish Oil Requirements: Take at least 2.5 grams of EPA and DHA sometime during the day. Take more according to the guidelines in chapter 9 if you have the complications associated with Toxic Fat Syndrome.

Day 6

BREAKFAST
> Vegetable Omelet

Ingredients for women	*Ingredients for men*
1 diced tomato	1 diced tomato
3/4 cup diced onions	3/4 cup diced onions
Chopped mushrooms, to taste	Chopped mushrooms, to taste
1 teaspoon olive oil	1 1/3 teaspoons olive oil
1 cup steamed asparagus tips	1 cup steamed asparagus tips
1 large whole egg, plus	1 large whole egg, plus
4 large egg whites or 1/2 cup egg substitute	6 large egg whites or 3/4 cup egg substitute
1/3 cup mandarin oranges	2/3 cup mandarin oranges

Sauté tomatoes, onions, and mushrooms in olive oil. Steam asparagus tips until tender. Beat eggs, adding 1 tablespoon of milk if desired. Add eggs to sautéed vegetables. Cook eggs on medium-low heat in olive oil until eggs are almost set. Lift edge of omelet with spatula to let liquid drain to the bottom. Place asparagus tips on top of omelet and fold over. Continue cooking until eggs are done. Garnish with mandarin oranges.

LUNCH
> Vegetarian Chili

Ingredients for women	Ingredients for men
1 cup soy protein crumbles (3 ounces ground turkey may be substituted)	1$^1/_2$ cups soy protein crumbles (4$^1/_2$ ounces ground turkey may be substituted)
1 teaspoon olive oil	1$^1/_3$ teaspoons olive oil
Onions, garlic, pepper, and mushrooms, chopped to taste	Onions, garlic, pepper, and mushrooms, chopped to taste
1 cup stewed tomatoes with liquid	1 cup stewed tomatoes with liquid
$^1/_4$ cup canned kidney beans, drained and rinsed	$^1/_2$ cup canned kidney beans, drained and rinsed
Chili powder to taste	Chili powder to taste
1 ounce reduced-fat cheese, shredded	1 ounce reduced-fat cheese, shredded

Sauté the crumbles (or ground turkey) in oil with the chopped onion, garlic, pepper, and mushrooms. Add tomatoes, kidney beans, and chili powder. Simmer for ten minutes. Top with cheese.

Late-Afternoon Zone Snack

DINNER
> Salsa Chicken

Ingredients for women	Ingredients for men
3 ounces boneless, skinless chicken breast	4 ounces boneless, skinless chicken breast
1/2 cup salsa (temperature of your choice)	1/2 cup salsa (temperature of your choice)
Sprinkling of low-fat cheese	Sprinkling of low-fat cheese
3 tablespoons guacamole	4 tablespoons guacamole
1 1/2 cups green beans, steamed, with salt to taste	1 1/2 cups green beans, steamed, with salt to taste
1/2 apple	1 apple

Preheat oven to 350 degrees. Put chicken in oven-proof dish, pour salsa on top, and sprinkle on cheese. Put in oven for approximately forty minutes. Top with guacamole. Serve green beans and apple (or another fruit) on the side.

Late-Evening Zone Snack

Fish Oil Requirements: Take at least 2.5 grams of EPA and DHA sometime during the day. Take more according to the guidelines in chapter 9 if you have the complications associated with Toxic Fat Syndrome.

Day 7

BREAKFAST

> Frozen Blueberry Yogurt

Ingredients for women

$1/2$ cup low-fat, plain yogurt

1 cup frozen blueberries

$1/2$ cup cottage cheese

1 tablespoon slivered almonds

1 teaspoon fructose, optional

Ingredients for men

1 cup low-fat, plain yogurt

1 cup frozen blueberries

$1/2$ cup cottage cheese

4 teaspoons slivered almonds

1 teaspoon fructose, optional

Put all in a food processor. Blend until smooth.

LUNCH

> Caprese Salad

Ingredients for women

2 tomatoes, sliced

3 ounces low-fat mozzarella cheese

1 clove garlic, minced

1 tablespoon chopped fresh
   basil leaves

1 teaspoon olive oil

Balsamic vinegar to taste

1 cup grapes

Ingredients for men

2 tomatoes, sliced

4 ounces low-fat mozzarella cheese

1 clove garlic, minced

1 tablespoon chopped fresh
   basil leaves

$1^1/3$ teaspoons olive oil

Balsamic vinegar to taste

$1^1/2$ cups grapes

Put sliced tomatoes on a plate. Top with cheese. Mix garlic, basil, and olive oil and put on top of tomatoes and cheese. Sprinkle with balsamic vinegar. Have grapes for dessert.

Late-Afternoon Zone Snack

DINNER
> Ten-Minute Fish Dish

Ingredients for women	Ingredients for men
4$^1/_2$-ounce fish fillet	6-ounce fish fillet
Salt and pepper	Salt and pepper
Lemon juice	Lemon juice
3 cups zucchini, rough chopped	3 cups zucchini, rough chopped
$^3/_4$ cup rough chopped onion	$^3/_4$ cup rough chopped onion
1 teaspoon olive oil	1$^1/_3$ teaspoons olive oil
1 cup strawberries	1 cup blueberries

Season fish with salt, black pepper, and fresh lemon juice, and sauté five minutes on each side until fish flakes. Put the onion and zucchini in a bowl, add the olive oil, salt, and pepper, and sauté until done. Place fish onto a plate, add vegetables and juice on top. Have fruit for dessert.

Late-Evening Zone Snack

Fish Oil Requirements: Take at least 2.5 grams of EPA and DHA sometime during the day. Take more according to the guidelines in chapter 9 if you have the complications associated with Toxic Fat Syndrome.

WEEK 3: Day 1

BREAKFAST
> Zone Muesli

Ingredients for women	Ingredients for men
$^1/_2$ cup low-fat cottage cheese	$^3/_4$ cup low-fat cottage cheese
7 grams protein powder	7 grams protein powder
$^1/_3$ cup rolled oats	$^1/_3$ cup rolled oats

3 canned apricots, chopped

1 tablespoon slivered almonds

3 canned apricots, chopped

4 teaspoons slivered almonds

Mix into a bowl and enjoy.

Note: You can easily alter the recipe by:

➤ Adding 1 block of fresh fruit rather than the apricots

➤ Increasing the cottage cheese by $1/4$ cup and omitting the protein powder

➤ Making the mixture ahead (without adding the nuts) and storing in the fridge so that it's ready each morning. (You can also double the recipe so that you have breakfast waiting in your refrigerator.) Just stir in the nuts before you eat it.

LUNCH

> Tuna and Three Bean Salad

Ingredients for women

3 ounces canned tuna

$1/4$ cup canned kidney beans, drained and rinsed

$1/4$ cup canned garbanzo beans, drained and rinsed

$1/4$ cup canned black beans, drained and rinsed

1 teaspoon olive oil

Rice vinegar to taste

1 teaspoon onion powder (or to taste)

$1/4$ teaspoon garlic powder (or to taste)

Bed of lettuce

Ingredients for men

4 ounces canned tuna

$1/4$ cup canned kidney beans, drained and rinsed

$1/4$ cup canned garbanzo beans, drained and rinsed

$1/4$ cup canned black beans, drained and rinsed

$1 1/3$ teaspoons olive oil

Rice vinegar to taste

1 teaspoon onion powder (or to taste)

$1/4$ teaspoon garlic powder (or to taste)

Bed of lettuce

$1/2$ apple (for dessert)

Mix together tuna and beans. Whisk together olive oil, rice vinegar, onion powder, and garlic powder. Pour over tuna mixture and toss. Serve over a bed of lettuce.

Late-Afternoon Zone Snack

DINNER
> Vegetable Stir-Fry

Ingredients for women	Ingredients for men
1 teaspoon olive oil	1$^{1}/_{3}$ teaspoons olive oil
3 ounces of skinless chicken breasts in thin strips	4 ounces of skinless chicken breasts in thin strips
1$^{1}/_{2}$ cups onions, minced	1$^{1}/_{2}$ cups onions, minced
1 clove garlic	1 clove garlic
2 cups broccoli florets	2 cups broccoli florets
2 cups mushrooms, thinly sliced	2 cups mushrooms, thiny sliced
$^{1}/_{2}$ cup grapes	1 cup grapes

Heat olive oil in a nonstick pan or wok over medium heat. Add chicken and stir until coated with oil. Add onions, garlic, broccoli, and mushrooms. Reduce heat to medium and continue to stir-fry until chicken is done and vegetables are just tender. Have grapes for dessert.

Late-Evening Zone Snack

Fish Oil Requirements: Take at least 2.5 grams of EPA and DHA sometime during the day. Take more according to the guidelines in chapter 9 if you have the complications associated with Toxic Fat Syndrome.

Day 2

BREAKFAST
> Yogurt-Topped Apple

Ingredients for women	*Ingredients for men*
1 apple, cored and halved lengthwise	1 apple, cored and halved lengthwise
1/2 cup plain low-fat yogurt	1 cup plain low-fat yogurt
1/8 teaspoon nutmeg	1/8 teaspoon nutmeg
1/8 teaspoon orange zest	1/8 teaspoon orange zest
1/8 teaspoon cinnamon	1/8 teaspoon cinnamon
1/2 cup low-fat cottage cheese	1/2 cup low-fat cottage cheese
1 tablespoon slivered almonds	4 teaspoons slivered almonds

Place apple cut side up in a small, microwavable dish. Cook apple in microwave set on high for four to five minutes. In a small mixing bowl, combine yogurt, nutmeg, orange zest, and cinnamon. Place cottage cheese in a serving dish. Sprinkle with almonds. When the apple is cooked (slightly soft), place apple on top of cottage cheese. Top with yogurt and serve.

LUNCH
> Grilled Shrimp Salad

Ingredients for women	*Ingredients for men*
Bed of green-leaf or romaine lettuce	Bed of green-leaf or romaine lettuce
1 cup broccoli, steamed until just tender	1 cup broccoli, steamed until just tender
1/2 green pepper	1/2 green pepper
1/4 cup canned kidney beans, drained and rinsed	1/4 cup canned kidney beans, drained and rinsed

1 medium tomato, sliced	1 medium tomato, sliced
1 teaspoon olive oil with vinegar to taste	$1^{1}/_{3}$ teaspoons olive oil with vinegar to taste
1 tablespoon lemon juice	1 tablespoon lemon juice
1 teaspoon Worcestershire sauce	1 teaspoon Worcestershire sauce
$^{1}/_{2}$ teaspoon ground pepper	$^{1}/_{2}$ teaspoon ground pepper
$4^{1}/_{2}$ ounces cooked shrimp	6 ounces cooked shrimp
$^{1}/_{2}$ pear	1 pear

Mix vegetables together. Whisk together olive oil, vinegar, lemon juice, Worcestershire sauce, and pepper. Pour over lettuce and toss. Put shrimp on top. Have pear for dessert.

Late-Afternoon Zone Snack

DINNER
> Salmon Patties

Ingredients for women	Ingredients for men
3 ounces canned pink salmon	$4^{1}/_{2}$ ounces canned pink salmon
2 egg whites	2 egg whites
$^{1}/_{3}$ cup slow-cooking oatmeal, cooked	$^{1}/_{3}$ cup slow-cooking oatmeal, cooked
$^{1}/_{4}$ onion, diced	$^{1}/_{4}$ onion, diced
1 teaspoon dill	1 teaspoon dill
Garlic salt and pepper	Garlic salt and pepper
1 teaspoon olive oil	$1^{1}/_{3}$ teaspoons olive oil
1 apple	$1^{1}/_{2}$ apples

Flake up salmon in a medium bowl. Combine all ingredients except olive oil and mix well with hands. Heat olive oil in pan at medium heat. Shape mixture into a patty and cook for about three to five minutes on each side (or until golden brown). Serve immediately. Have apple for dessert.

Late-Evening Zone Snack

Fish Oil Requirements: Take at least 2.5 grams of EPA and DHA sometime during the day. Take more according to the guidelines in chapter 9 if you have the complications associated with Toxic Fat Syndrome.

DAY 3

BREAKFAST
> Salsa Scramble

Ingredients for women	*Ingredients for men*
4 egg whites or $1/2$ cup egg substitute	6 egg whites or $3/4$ cup egg substitute
$2/3$ teaspoon olive oil	1 teaspoon olive oil
$1/4$ cup canned black beans, drained and rinsed	$1/4$ cup canned black beans, drained and rinsed
$1^1/2$ cups onions	$1^1/2$ cups onions
$1/2$ cup salsa	$1/2$ cup salsa
1 tablespoon guacamole	1 tablespoon guacamole
1 ounce shredded low-fat mozzarella cheese	1 ounce shredded low-fat mozzarella cheese
	$3/4$ cup V8 juice

Crack eggs and separate yolk from whites, or use egg substitute. Set aside. Heat nonstick skillet and add olive oil. Heat black beans in microwave until warm. Sauté onions in olive oil until tender. Add eggs to onions and scramble. Place egg mixture on plate. Mix salsa with beans. Place mixture on top of eggs. Top with cheese. If needed, put plate in microwave for 20 seconds to melt cheese. Place guacamole on top of cheese. Men have V8 on the side.

LUNCH
> Bacon and Apple Sandwich

Ingredients for women	Ingredients for men
1 slice rye bread	1 slice rye bread
1 tablespoon natural peanut butter	4 teaspoons natural peanut butter
3 ounces lean Canadian bacon	4 ounces lean Canadian bacon
1/2 apple, thinly sliced	1 apple, thinly sliced
1/2 cup alfalfa sprouts, optional	1/2 cup alfalfa sprouts, optional

Lightly toast bread and spread with peanut butter. Layer Canadian bacon, apple, and sprouts.

Late-Afternoon Zone Snack

DINNER
> Broccoli Casserole

Ingredients for women	Ingredients for men
2 cups chopped broccoli	2 cups chopped broccoli
2 cups chopped mushrooms	2 cups chopped mushrooms
3/4 cup chopped onions	3/4 cup chopped onions
1 cup chopped peppers	1 cup chopped peppers
1/4 cup canned chickpeas, drained and rinsed	1/2 cup canned chickpeas, drained and rinsed

¹/₂ cup egg substitute	³/₄ cup egg substitute
1 ounce low-fat mozzarella cheese	1 ounce low-fat mozzarella cheese
1 teaspoon light mayonnaise	1 teaspoon light mayonnaise
2 teaspoons slivered almonds	1 tablespoon slivered almonds

Put veggies in a large casserole pan. Mix egg substitute, cheese, and mayo. Pour over vegetables. Sprinkle almonds over the top. Bake at 350 degrees for thirty-five to forty minutes.

Late-Evening Zone Snack

Fish Oil Requirements: Take at least 2.5 grams of EPA and DHA sometime during the day. Take more according to the guidelines in chapter 9 if you have the complications associated with Toxic Fat Syndrome.

Day 4

BREAKFAST
> Fruit Smoothie

Ingredients for women	*Ingredients for men*
14 grams protein powder	21 grams protein powder
1 cup low-fat milk	1 cup low-fat milk
¹/₂ cup blueberries	1 cup blueberries
1 cup strawberries	1 cup strawberries
3 macadamia nuts, crushed	4 macadamia nuts, crushed
6 ice cubes	6 ice cubes

Place all ingredients, except nuts, in a blender and blend at high speed until smooth. Top with crushed nuts.

LUNCH
> Nicoise Salad

Ingredients for women

1 small Red Bliss potato,
   cooked, sliced

1$\frac{1}{2}$ cups green beans, ends
   removed, cooked, halved

Bed of red-leaf or green-leaf lettuce

$\frac{1}{4}$ medium cucumber, peeled,
   quartered, thinly sliced

$\frac{1}{2}$ tomato, cut into wedges

$\frac{1}{2}$ cup small sweet onion (Vidalia),
   sliced into thin rings

2 hard-boiled eggs, quartered,
   yolks removed

2 ounces albacore tuna packed
   in water, drained

1 teaspoon olive oil and vinegar
   to taste

Ingredients for men

1 small Red Bliss potato,
   cooked, sliced

1$\frac{1}{2}$ cups green beans, ends
   removed, cooked, halved

Bed of red-leaf or green-leaf lettuce

$\frac{1}{4}$ medium cucumber, peeled,
   quartered, thinly sliced

$\frac{1}{2}$ tomato, cut into wedges

$\frac{1}{2}$ cup small sweet onion (Vidalia),
   sliced into thin rings

2 hard-boiled eggs, quartered,
   yolks removed

3 ounces albacore tuna packed
   in water, drained

1$\frac{1}{3}$ teaspoons olive oil and vinegar
   to taste

$\frac{1}{2}$ pear for dessert

Gently toss all ingredients in salad bowl; add dressing.

Late-Afternoon Zone Snack

DINNER
> Easy Barbeque Tofu and Vegetables

Ingredients for women	Ingredients for men
2 stalks celery	2 stalks celery
3/4 cup onion, diced	3/4 cup onion, diced
1 teaspoon olive oil	1 1/3 teaspoons olive oil
1 clove garlic, minced	1 clove garlic, minced
1 red or green pepper, diced	1 red or green pepper, diced
6 ounces firm tofu, cubed	8 ounces firm tofu, cubed
1/2 cup vegetable broth	1/2 cup vegetable broth
1 teaspoon apple cider vinegar	1 teaspoon apple cider vinegar
2 tablespoons prepared barbeque sauce	2 tablespoons prepared barbeque sauce
1 teaspoon prepared mustard	1 teaspoon prepared mustard
1/2 cup grapes	1 cup grapes

Sauté onions and celery in olive oil over medium-high heat until onions are soft and translucent. Add garlic, green pepper, and tofu and sauté three to five minutes. Add remaining ingredients and stir. Simmer covered about twenty minutes. Have fruit for dessert.

Late-Evening Zone Snack

Fish Oil Requirements: Take at least 2.5 grams of EPA and DHA sometime during the day. Take more according to the guidelines in chapter 9 if you have the complications associated with Toxic Fat Syndrome.

Day 5

BREAKFAST

> Cottage Cheese with Raspberry Sauce

Ingredients for women	Ingredients for men
3/4 cup low-fat cottage cheese	1 cup low-fat cottage cheese
1/4 cup blueberries	1/2 cup blueberries
1/2 cup canned peaches in water, drained	1/2 cup canned peaches in water, drained
1/4 cup grapes	1/2 cup grapes
1 cup raspberries and 1 tablespoon water	1 cup raspberries and 1 tablespoon water
1 tablespoon slivered almonds	4 teaspoons slivered almonds

Mound cottage cheese in the center of a serving plate. Arrange blueberries, peaches, and grapes around cottage cheese. Place raspberries in a blender and puree. Pour pureed raspberries over cottage cheese and fruit. Sprinkle with nuts.

LUNCH

> Turkey Burger with Cheese

Ingredients for women	Ingredients for men
3 ounces ground turkey	4 1/2 ounces ground turkey
Salt and pepper to taste	Salt and pepper to taste
1 ounce reduced-fat cheese	1 ounce reduced-fat cheese
1 tablespoon light mayonnaise	1 tablespoon light mayonnaise
1/2 hamburger bun	1/2 hamburger bun
1 large lettuce leaf	1 large lettuce leaf
1 thick tomato slice	1 thick tomato slice

1 dill pickle wedge, optional
2/3 cup unsweetened applesauce
    sprinkled with cinnamon

1 dill pickle wedge, optional
1 cup unsweetened applesauce
    sprinkled with cinnamon
6 peanuts on the side

Cook burger in nonstick skillet until medium with salt and pepper to taste. Top with cheese. Spread mayo on bun and top with lettuce, burger, and tomato. Serve with pickle. Have applesauce for dessert.

Late-Afternoon Zone Snack

DINNER
> Ginger Pork

Ingredients for women
2 teaspoons soy sauce
1 teaspoon mirin (or 1 teaspoon sake
    and a pinch of sugar), optional
1 teaspoon sesame oil
1 teaspoon fresh gingerroot, grated
3 ounces pork, sliced in thin strips
1 teaspoon garlic, minced
1/4 teaspoon caraway seeds, ground
4 cups cabbage, shredded
1/2 cup chicken stock
2/3 cup unsweetened applesauce

Ingredients for men
2 teaspoons soy sauce
1 teaspoon mirin (or 1 teaspoon sake
    and a pinch of sugar), optional
1 1/2 teaspoons sesame oil
1 teaspoon fresh gingerroot, grated
4 ounces pork, sliced in thin strips
1 teaspoon garlic, minced
1/4 teaspoon caraway seeds, ground
4 cups cabbage, shredded
1/2 cup chicken stock
1 cup unsweetened applesauce

In a bowl, make sauce by combining soy sauce, mirin, sesame oil, and grated ginger. Marinate pork strips in sauce for two minutes. Spray nonstick pan with vegetable spray. Remove pork from marinade and sauté for one minute. Reduce heat to medium and add garlic, caraway seeds, and cabbage. Cover and simmer in chicken stock until cabbage is tender. Have applesauce for dessert.

Late-Evening Zone Snack

Fish Oil Requirements: Take at least 2.5 grams of EPA and DHA sometime during the day. Take more according to the guidelines in chapter 9 if you have the complications associated with Toxic Fat Syndrome.

Day 6

BREAKFAST
> Chicken and Chickpea Hash

Ingredients for women	*Ingredients for men*
1 teaspoon olive oil	$1^{1}/_{3}$ teaspoons olive oil
$4^{1}/_{2}$ ounces ground chicken	6 ounces ground chicken
$3/_4$ cup onion, diced	$3/_4$ cup onion, diced
2 cups mushrooms, diced	2 cups mushrooms, diced
$1/_3$ cup boiled potato, mashed (without butter or milk)	$1/_3$ cup boiled potato, mashed (without butter or milk)
$1/_4$ cup canned chickpeas, drained, rinsed, and mashed	$1/_4$ cup canned chickpeas, drained, rinsed, and mashed
$1/_8$ teaspoon Worcestershire sauce	$1/_8$ teaspoon Worcestershire sauce
$1/_8$ teaspoon lemon herb seasoning	$1/_8$ teaspoon lemon herb seasoning
$1/_8$ teaspoon chili powder	$1/_8$ teaspoon chili powder
Paprika and parsley for garnish	Paprika and parsley for garnish
	1 tangerine (for dessert)

In a medium nonstick sauté pan, heat oil. Sauté chicken, onion, and mushrooms until chicken is cooked. Add remaining ingredients (except paprika and parsley) and cook on medium-high heat until browned, about three to five minutes. Place on a serving dish. Garnish with paprika and parsley.

LUNCH
> Miso Soup with Tofu

Ingredients for women	Ingredients for men
6 ounces firm tofu	8 ounces firm tofu
$1/2$ cup green onions	$1/2$ cup green onions
1 tablespoon miso	1 tablespoon miso
1 cup vegetable stock	1 cup vegetable stock
1 cup mandarin oranges	$1^1/3$ cups mandarin oranges

Cut the tofu into cubes. Slice the green onions diagonally. Heat vegetable stock for three to four minutes and gently dissolve the miso in the soup. Add the tofu and heat it gently, taking care that stock doesn't come to a boil. Garnish with spring onion just before serving. Have mandarin oranges for dessert.

Late-Afternoon Zone Snack

DINNER
> Italian-Style Chicken

Ingredients for women	Ingredients for men
3 ounces chicken tenderloin, sliced diagonally	4 ounces chicken tenderloin, sliced diagonally

1¹/₂ cups onion, chopped	1¹/₂ cups onion, chopped
¹/₂ teaspoon Worcestershire sauce	¹/₂ teaspoon Worcestershire sauce
¹/₄ cup chickpeas, rinsed	¹/₂ cup chickpeas, rinsed, drained
1¹/₂ cups plum tomatoes, chopped	1¹/₂ cups plum tomatoes, chopped
3 cups spinach, chopped	3 cups spinach, chopped
1 teaspoon olive oil	1¹/₃ teaspoons olive oil
¹/₂ cup chicken stock	¹/₂ cup chicken stock
1 teaspoon garlic, chopped	1 teaspoon garlic, chopped
1¹/₂ teaspoons dried oregano	1¹/₂ teaspoons dried oregano
Salt and pepper, to taste	Salt and pepper, to taste

In a medium nonstick sauté pan, heat ²/₃ teaspoon of the oil. Add chicken, ¹/₂ cup of the onion, and Worcestershire sauce. In a second nonstick sauté pan, heat remaining oil. Stir in 1 cup onion, chickpeas, plum tomatoes, spinach, stock, garlic, oregano, and salt and pepper. Sauté until spinach begins to wilt. Place vegetable mixture on serving plate and top with chicken.

Late-Evening Zone Snack

Fish Oil Requirements: Take at least 2.5 grams of EPA and DHA sometime during the day. Take more according to the guidelines in chapter 9 if you have the complications associated with Toxic Fat Syndrome.

Day 7

BREAKFAST

> Scrambled Eggs with Blueberry Orange Salad

Ingredients for women
²/₃ teaspoon olive oil

Ingredients for men
1 teaspoon olive oil

1 soy sausage (7 grams of protein)
Onions and peppers, chopped,
    about 1/4 cup each
1/2 cup egg substitute
1 cup blueberries
1/2 orange, sectioned
2 teaspoons lime juice
6 peanuts, chopped

1 soy sausage (7 grams of protein)
Onions and peppers, chopped,
    about 1/4 cup each
2/3 cup egg substitute
1 cup blueberries
1 orange, sectioned
2 teaspoons lime juice
6 peanuts, chopped

Heat oil in a nonstick pan on medium-high heat. Add sausage, onions, and peppers. Cook until onions are translucent. Add eggs and scramble until eggs are firm. Mix blueberries, orange, lime juice, and nuts together for the salad.

LUNCH
> Crab Bisque

Ingredients for women
3/4 cup chopped onion
1 teaspoon olive oil
1 teaspoon cornstarch
1 cup skim or 1 percent milk
3 ounces canned crabmeat
    (other seafood may be used),
    21 grams of protein
Salt and pepper to taste
Paprika as a garnish, optional
1/2 cup grapes

Ingredients for men
3/4 cup chopped onion
1 1/3 teaspoons olive oil
1 teaspoon cornstarch
1 cup skim or 1 percent milk
4 ounces canned crabmeat
    (other seafood may be used),
    28 grams of protein
Salt and pepper to taste
Paprika as a garnish, optional
1 cup grapes

Sauté onion in olive oil until soft and translucent. Mix cornstarch in cold milk and then add to onion. Heat and stir until thickened slightly. Add salt and pepper. Stir in crab and heat through. Garnish with paprika. Have grapes for dessert.

Late-Afternoon Zone Snack

DINNER
> Stir-Fry Salmon with Snow Peas

Ingredients for women	Ingredients for men
1 teaspoon olive oil	$1^1/_3$ teaspoons olive oil
3 ounces canned salmon	$4^1/_2$ ounces canned salmon
1 whole egg	1 whole egg
$^1/_2$ cup salsa*	$^1/_2$ cup salsa*
1 teaspoon dill	1 teaspoon dill
$^3/_4$ cup onion, chopped	$^3/_4$ cup onion, chopped
$^1/_2$ cup fresh snow peas	$^1/_2$ cup fresh snow peas
$^1/_3$ cup water chestnuts, sliced	$^1/_3$ cup water chestnuts, sliced
1 cup mushrooms, sliced	1 cup mushrooms, sliced
1 teaspoon Worcestershire sauce	1 teaspoon Worcestershire sauce
1 tablespoon balsamic vinegar	1 tablespoon balsamic vinegar
$^1/_8$ teaspoon celery seed	$^1/_8$ teaspoon celery seed
$^1/_8$ teaspoon dry ground double superfine mustard	$^1/_8$ teaspoon dry ground double superfine mustard
	$^1/_2$ pear (for dessert)

Heat $^2/_3$ teaspoon oil in a medium nonstick sauté pan. Combine salmon, egg, salsa, and dill. Sauté until heated through. Heat remaining oil in a second nonstick pan. Add onion, snow peas, water chestnuts, mushrooms, Worcestershire sauce, vinegar, celery seed, and mustard. Sauté until vegetables are tender. Combine salmon mixture with vegetables and serve.

Note: We used a medium-heat salsa. Use whatever strength you prefer.

Late-Evening Zone Snack

Fish Oil Requirements: Take at least 2.5 grams of EPA and DHA sometime during the day. Take more according to the guidelines in chapter 9 if you have the complications associated with Toxic Fat Syndrome.

WEEK 4: Day 1

BREAKFAST
> Fruit Compote

Ingredients for women	*Ingredients for men*
3/4 cup low-fat cottage cheese	1 cup low-fat cottage cheese
1/2 teaspoon cinnamon	1/2 teaspoon cinnamon
1/8 teaspoon nutmeg	1/8 teaspoon nutmeg
1 teaspoon orange zest	1 teaspoon orange zest
1 tablespoon almonds, slivered and toasted	4 teaspoons almonds, slivered and toasted
1/2 Granny Smith apple, cored and chopped	1 Granny Smith apple, cored and chopped
1/2 grapefruit in sections	1/2 grapefruit in sections
1/3 cup mandarin orange sections	1/3 cup mandarin orange sections
Paprika as garnish	Paprika as garnish

In a small mixing bowl, combine cottage cheese with cinnamon, nutmeg, and orange zest. Mound into serving dish. Combine almonds, apple pieces, grapefruit, and orange sections, and spoon over cheese. Sprinkle paprika over cottage cheese and serve.

LUNCH
> Cilantro Egg Salad

Ingredients for women	Ingredients for men
3/4 cup egg substitute	1 cup egg substitute
1 tablespoon reduced-fat mayonnaise	4 teaspoons reduced-fat mayonnaise
1/8 teaspoon dry mustard	1/8 teaspoon dry mustard
1/2 teaspoon garlic, minced	1/2 teaspoon garlic, minced
1/8 teaspoon cilantro	1/8 teaspoon cilantro
Salt and pepper to taste	Salt and pepper to taste
1/4 cup celery, minced	1/4 cup celery, minced
3/4 cup canned mushrooms, drained, diced	3/4 cup canned mushrooms, drained, diced
1/3 cup onion, chopped	1/3 cup onion, chopped
1/4 cup kidney beans	1/4 cup kidney beans
3/4 cup cucumber, peeled and sliced	3/4 cup cucumber, peeled and sliced
1/3 cup tomatoes, diced	1/3 cup tomatoes, diced
Bed of lettuce	Bed of lettuce
1/2 cup grapes	1 cup grapes

Pour egg substitute into a ten-ounce microwave-safe dish and cook on high (100 percent) setting for one to two-and-a-half minutes, or until set. Push cooked egg portions to center of the dish and continue cooking in 30-second intervals on high setting. When done, cool and dice cooked egg substitute. In a small bowl, blend mayonnaise and seasonings. Combine cooked egg substitute with the other ingredients in a medium bowl. Toss to coat with mayonnaise and serve on a bed of lettuce. Have grapes for dessert.

Late-Afternoon Zone Snack

DINNER
> Sautéed Green Beans with Tofu

Ingredients for women	*Ingredients for men*
1 teaspoon olive oil, divided	1$1/3$ teaspoons olive oil, divided
6 ounces extra-firm tofu, 1-inch	8 ounces extra-firm tofu, 1-inch
$1/2$ teaspoon Worcestershire sauce	$1/2$ teaspoon Worcestershire sauce
$1/8$ teaspoon celery salt	$1/8$ teaspoon celery salt
1$1/2$ cups green beans, trimmed, 2-inch pieces	1$1/2$ cups green beans, trimmed, 2-inch pieces
$1/2$ cup onion, chopped	$1/2$ cup onion, chopped
$1/2$ teaspoon garlic, minced	$1/2$ teaspoon garlic, minced
2 teaspoons cider vinegar	2 teaspoons cider vinegar
$1/8$ teaspoon nutmeg	$1/8$ teaspoon nutmeg
$1/8$ teaspoon cinnamon	$1/8$ teaspoon cinnamon
$1/8$ teaspoon lemon herb seasoning	$1/8$ teaspoon lemon herb seasoning
$1/8$ teaspoon ground double superfine mustard	$1/8$ teaspoon ground double superfine mustard
$1/2$ teaspoon soy sauce	$1/2$ teaspoon soy sauce
Salt and pepper to taste	Salt and pepper to taste
1 apple (for dessert)	1 apple and 1 plum (for dessert)

Heat ²/₃ teaspoon oil in medium nonstick sauté pan. Gently mix tofu, Worcestershire sauce, and celery salt. Stir-fry until tofu is browned and crusted on all sides. In a second nonstick sauté pan, heat remaining oil and add in green beans, onion, garlic, vinegar, nutmeg, cinnamon, lemon herb seasoning, mustard, soy sauce, and salt and pepper. Cook until beans are tender-crisp. Place beans on serving plate and top with tofu.

Late-Evening Zone Snack

Fish Oil Requirements: Take at least 2.5 grams of EPA and DHA sometime during the day. Take more according to the guidelines in chapter 9 if you have the complications associated with Toxic Fat Syndrome.

Day 2

BREAKFAST
> **Yogurt with Blueberries and Almonds**

Ingredients for women	*Ingredients for men*
1 cup plain, low-fat yogurt	1 cup plain, low-fat yogurt
¹/₂ cup blueberries	1 cup blueberries
1 tablespoon almonds	4 teaspoons almonds
1 ounce Canadian bacon or 3 turkey bacon strips	2 ounces Canadian bacon or 6 turkey bacon strips

Mix together and enjoy. Serve bacon on the side.

LUNCH
> Taco Burger

Ingredients for women	Ingredients for men
3 ounces lean (90 percent fat-free) ground beef	4^1/$_2$ ounces lean (90 percent fat-free) ground beef
^{1}/$_2$ cup salsa	1 cup salsa
1 teaspoon olive oil	1^1/$_3$ teaspoons olive oil
^{1}/$_4$ cup black beans, rinsed	^{1}/$_4$ cup black beans, rinsed
^{1}/$_2$ teaspoon garlic, minced	^{1}/$_2$ teaspoon garlic, minced
Onion, chopped, about 2 tablespoons	Onion, chopped, about 2 tablespoons
^{1}/$_2$ teaspoon Worcestershire sauce	^{1}/$_2$ teaspoon Worcestershire sauce
^{1}/$_2$ teaspoon celery salt	^{1}/$_2$ teaspoon celery salt
1 tablespoon lemon- or lime-flavored water, optional	1 tablespoon lemon- or lime-flavored water, optional
1 ounce low-fat Monterrey Jack cheese, shredded	1 ounce low-fat Monterrey Jack cheese, shredded
Lettuce, shredded	Lettuce, shredded
5 taco chips, crushed	5 taco chips, crushed

In a small bowl, combine ground beef and ^{1}/$_4$ cup salsa. Form into patty. Heat ^{1}/$_2$ teaspoon oil in a medium nonstick pan and sauté patty, turning until cooked through. In a second nonstick sauté pan, heat remaining oil. Place beans, garlic, ^{1}/$_4$ cup salsa, onion, Worcestershire sauce, celery salt, and water in the second pan. Cook until heated through. Put lettuce onto a plate. Add patty, sprinkle with taco chips, and top with bean mixture and cheese.

Late-Afternoon Zone Snack

DINNER
> Ginger Chicken

Ingredients for women
1 teaspoon olive oil
3 ounces boneless, skinless
    chicken breast, cut into strips
2 cups broccoli florets
1 1/2 cups snow peas
3/4 cup yellow onion, peeled and
    chopped
1 teaspoon fresh ginger, grated
1/4 cup water
1/2 cup grapes

Ingredients for men
1 1/3 teaspoons olive oil
4 ounces boneless, skinless
    chicken breast, cut into strips
2 cups broccoli florets
1 1/2 cups snow peas
3/4 cup yellow onion, peeled and
    chopped
1 teaspoon fresh ginger, grated
1/4 cup water
1 cup grapes

In a wok or large nonstick pan, heat oil over medium-high heat. Add chicken and sauté, turning frequently, until lightly browned, about five minutes. Add broccoli, snow peas, onion, ginger, and water. Continue cooking, stirring often, until chicken is done, water is reduced to a glaze, and vegetables are tender, about twenty minutes. If the pan dries out during cooking, add water in tablespoon increments to keep moist. Serve grapes for dessert, or garnish dish with grapes.

Late-Evening Zone Snack

Fish Oil Requirements: Take at least 2.5 grams of EPA and DHA sometime during the day. Take more according to the guidelines in chapter 9 if you have the complications associated with Toxic Fat Syndrome.

Day 3

BREAKFAST

> Apple and Cheese Melt

Ingredients for women	Ingredients for men
$1/4$ cup water	$1/4$ cup water
$1/4$ teaspoon powdered cinnamon	$1/4$ teaspoon powdered cinnamon
1 tablespoon raisins	1 tablespoon raisins
1 apple, sliced	$1^1/2$ apples, sliced
3 ounces low-fat mozzarella	4 ounces low-fat mozzarella
1 tablespoon slivered almonds	4 teaspoons slivered almonds

Add water, cinnamon, and raisins to an 8- or 9-inch skillet with a lid. Wash apples; peel if desired. Halve apples and scoop out inner core with a teaspoon, grapefruit spoon, or melon baller. Slice and add to skillet. Cover and bring to boil. Reduce heat and simmer for about four to six minutes, until almost tender and water has evaporated. Grate cheese. Remove lid from skillet; sprinkle nuts, then cheese over fruit. Cover and simmer for two to three minutes until cheese melts, then remove from heat. Or simply sprinkle on cheese, cover, and remove from heat. Use a spatula to slide apple and cheese onto a plate. Serve immediately.

LUNCH

> Tuna Fruit Salad

Ingredients for women	Ingredients for men
2 tablespoons plain, low-fat yogurt	2 tablespoons plain, low-fat yogurt
$1/3$ teaspoon Dijon mustard	$1/3$ teaspoon Dijon mustard
$1/8$ teaspoon parsley flakes	$1/8$ teaspoon parsley flakes
$1/8$ teaspoon dill, dried	$1/8$ teaspoon dill, dried

Pinch of onion powder

Salt and pepper to taste

3 ounces chunk light tuna, drained

1 tablespoon celery, chopped fine

1 tablespoon slivered almonds, toasted

$1/2$ cup blueberries

1 cup strawberries, sliced

$1/2$ apple, chopped

Bed of romaine lettuce, chopped

Pinch of paprika for garnish

Pinch of onion powder

Salt and pepper to taste

4 ounces chunk light tuna, drained

1 tablespoon celery, chopped fine

4 teaspoons slivered almonds, toasted

1 cup blueberries

1 cup strawberries, sliced

$1/2$ apple, chopped

Bed of romaine lettuce, chopped

Pinch of paprika for garnish

Mix yogurt and spices in a bowl. Add tuna, celery, and almonds. In another bowl, mix fruit together. Place lettuce on a plate, and then place tuna mixture in the center. Surround with fruit salad. Sprinkle paprika on top of tuna salad.

Late-Afternoon Zone Snack

DINNER
> Baked Salmon

Ingredients for women

1 teaspoon olive oil

$3/4$ cup onions, sliced

1 cup asparagus spears

1 red bell pepper, cut in rings

$1/4$ cup canned chickpeas,
    drained and rinsed

1 clove garlic, minced

Ingredients for men

$1^{1}/_{3}$ teaspoons olive oil

$3/4$ cup onions, sliced

1 cup asparagus spears

1 red bell pepper, cut in rings

$1/4$ cup canned chickpeas,
    drained and rinsed

1 clove garlic, minced

1 tablespoon fresh dill	1 tablespoon fresh dill
1 tablespoon fresh chopped chives	1 tablespoon fresh chopped chives
$3/4$ cup water	$3/4$ cup water
Dash of hot sauce	Dash of hot sauce
$4^1/2$ ounces salmon	6 ounces salmon
Black pepper	Black pepper
Celery salt	Celery salt
$1/3$ tablespoon Dijon mustard	$1/3$ tablespoon Dijon mustard
	1 kiwi (for dessert)

Place oil in nonstick pan and sauté vegetables with garlic, dill, and chives on high heat for about two minutes. Add water and hot sauce and bring to a quick boil. Place vegetables in baking dish. Sprinkle the salmon with black pepper and celery salt. Spread Dijon mustard on top of salmon. Place salmon on bed of vegetables in pan. Bake uncovered in a 400-degree oven for fifteen to twenty minutes or until fish flakes. Garnish with more chives if desired.

Late-Evening Zone Snack

Fish Oil Requirements: Take at least 2.5 grams of EPA and DHA sometime during the day. Take more according to the guidelines in chapter 9 if you have the complications associated with Toxic Fat Syndrome.

Day 4

BREAKFAST
> Mandarin Orange Scramble

Ingredients for women	*Ingredients for men*
1 teaspoon olive oil	$1^1/3$ teaspoons olive oil

2 cups mushrooms, sliced	2 cups mushrooms, sliced
$3/4$ cup onion, chopped	$3/4$ cup onion, chopped
1 cup green pepper, cut in half and sliced	1 cup green pepper, cut in half and sliced
1 tablespoon balsamic vinegar	1 tablespoon balsamic vinegar
$1/2$ teaspoon Worcestershire sauce	$1/2$ teaspoon Worcestershire sauce
$1/4$ teaspoon celery salt	$1/4$ teaspoon celery salt
$1/4$ teaspoon dried dill	$1/4$ teaspoon dried dill
$3/4$ cup egg substitute	1 cup egg substitute
$3/4$ cup snow peas, julienned	$3/4$ cup snow peas, julienned
$1/3$ cup mandarin orange sections	$2/3$ cup mandarin orange sections
$1/4$ teaspoon lemon herb seasoning	$1/4$ teaspoon lemon herb seasoning

Heat oil in a medium, nonstick sauté pan. Sauté mushrooms, onion, peppers, vinegar, Worcestershire sauce, celery salt, and dill. Cook until the vegetables are crisp-tender, about five to seven minutes. Then pour in the egg substitute and snow peas. Cook, stirring, until set. Remove from the heat. Garnish late with mandarin orange sections. Sprinkle on lemon herb seasoning and serve.

LUNCH

> Vegetable Beef Soup

Ingredients for women	*Ingredients for men*
$4^{1}/2$ ounces lean ground beef	6 ounces lean ground beef
1 cup celery, diced fine	1 cup celery, diced fine
$1/2$ cup carrots, diced fine	$1/2$ cup carrots, diced fine
$3/4$ cup onion, diced fine	$3/4$ cup onion, diced fine
$3/4$ cup tomato, chopped	$3/4$ cup tomato, chopped

1/2 cup tomato puree	1 cup tomato puree
1 teaspoon olive oil	1 1/3 teaspoons olive oil
2 cups beef stock	2 cups beef stock
Salt and pepper to taste	Salt and pepper to taste
4 green peppercorns	4 green peppercorns
1 garlic clove, minced	1 garlic clove, minced
1/8 teaspoon marjoram	1/8 teaspoon marjoram
1/8 teaspoon Worcestershire sauce	1/8 teaspoon Worcestershire sauce
1/4 teaspoon chives	1/4 teaspoon chives
1 teaspoon parsley	1 teaspoon parsley
1/8 teaspoon oregano	1/8 teaspoon oregano

Combine all the ingredients in a large saucepan. Bring to a boil and then simmer for thirty-five to forty minutes, stirring occasionally until all vegetables are tender.

Late-Afternoon Zone Snack

DINNER
> Chicken Marinara with Three Bean Salad*

Ingredients for women

Ingredients for men

1 1/2 cups green beans, washed, ends removed, and cut in half	1 1/2 cups green beans, washed, ends removed, and cut in half
1/4 cup canned chickpeas, drained and rinsed	1/4 cup canned chickpeas, drained and rinsed
1/4 cup canned kidney beans, drained and rinsed	1/2 cup canned kidney beans, drained and rinsed
1 teaspoon olive oil	1 1/3 teaspoons olive oil

2 tablespoons cider vinegar (or to taste)	2 tablespoons cider vinegar (or to taste)
1 teaspoon dried chives	1 teaspoon dried chives
1 teaspoon dried parsley	1 teaspoon dried parsley
1/2 teaspoon freshly ground pepper or to taste	1/2 teaspoon freshly ground pepper or to taste
1 1/2 teaspoons dried basil	1 1/2 teaspoons dried basil
2 ounces boneless, skinless chicken breast	3 ounces boneless, skinless chicken breast
2 tablespoons prepared tomato sauce	2 tablespoons prepared tomato sauce
1/4 teaspoon garlic powder (or to taste)	1/4 teaspoon garlic powder (or to taste)
1 ounce low-fat mozzarella cheese	1 ounce low-fat mozzarella cheese

Preheat oven to 450 degrees. In a large pot fitted with a steaming basket, bring one inch water to boil. Add green beans to the basket and steam until tender-crisp, about ten minutes. Remove from basket, drain, and combine with chickpeas and kidney beans. In a small mixing bowl, combine olive oil, vinegar, chives, parsley, pepper, and one teaspoon of the basil; experiment with the oil-vinegar ratio to taste. Toss with beans, cover, and refrigerate for thirty minutes. Place chicken in a large piece of foil. Top chicken with tomato sauce and sprinkle with remaining 1/2 teaspoon basil, garlic powder, and cheese. Fold foil loosely over chicken, leaving ample space for air. Carefully turn up and seal the ends and the middle so that the juices won't leak out. Bake in the preheated oven for twenty minutes or until cooked through. Remove from oven and carefully open foil to prevent steam burns. Serve with bean salad.

*If possible, make the three-bean salad ahead of time (up to two days) and store tightly sealed in the refrigerator.

Late-Evening Zone Snack

Fish Oil Requirements: Take at least 2.5 grams of EPA and DHA sometime during the day. Take more according to the guidelines in chapter 9 if you have the complications associated with Toxic Fat Syndrome.

Day 5

BREAKFAST

> Overnight Eggnog Oatmeal

Ingredients for women	*Ingredients for men*
$2/3$ cup steel-cut oatmeal, cooked	1 cup steel-cut oatmeal, cooked
$1/8$ teaspoon sun-dried sea salt	$1/8$ teaspoon sun-dried sea salt
1 cup boiling water	1 cup boiling water
21 grams unsweetened protein powder	28 grams unsweetened protein powder
$1/8$ to $1/4$ teaspoon ground nutmeg	$1/8$ to $1/4$ teaspoon ground nutmeg
1 teaspoon pure vanilla extract	1 teaspoon pure vanilla extract
$1/4$ teaspoon white stevia extract powder or 4 drops stevia extract liquid	$1/4$ teaspoon white stevia extract powder or 4 drops stevia extract liquid
1 teaspoon almond or walnut oil (or 9 almonds or 3 macadamia nuts, raw or lightly toasted, chopped coarsely)	$1^{1}/3$ teaspoons almond or walnut oil (or 9 almonds or 3 macadamia nuts, raw or lightly toasted, chopped coarsely)
$1/2$ cup blueberries	$1/2$ cup blueberries

1. Add oats and sea salt to a wide-mouth thermos bottle. Add boiling water. Immediately cover tightly with a lid. Allow to sit overnight.

2. In the morning, stir thoroughly with a wide wooden spoon and transfer to a large cereal bowl. Add protein powder, nutmeg, vanilla, and

stevia. Stir well to dissolve lumps. Top with blueberries and oil or chopped nuts. Serve immediately or return to thermos bottle to serve later.

Variation (Crock-Pot cooking)

1. Just before bedtime, add oats and sea salt to a mini-Crock-Pot. (Do *not* use a large Crock-Pot for a small volume of cereal. Unit must be at least half full or too much water will evaporate during cooking.) Add cold water. Set dial to the lowest setting.

2. Cover and cook all night. In the morning, turn off heat. Let stand for ten to fifteen minutes. Stir thoroughly with a wooden spoon. Transfer to a large cereal bowl. Add protein powder, nutmeg, vanilla, and stevia. Stir well to dissolve lumps. If soy protein is used, you may need to add additional hot water, a few tablespoons at a time, to create a smooth mixture. Top with oil or chopped nuts. Serve immediately or transfer to thermos bottle to serve later.

LUNCH
> Tomato Basil Salad

Ingredients for women	Ingredients for men
Bed of romaine lettuce, chopped	Bed of romaine lettuce, chopped
1/4 cup chickpeas, rinsed and finely chopped	1/2 cup chickpeas, rinsed and finely chopped
1 tablespoon fresh parsley, chopped	1 tablespoon fresh parsley, chopped
1 teaspoon olive oil	1 1/3 teaspoons olive oil
1 tablespoon red wine vinegar	1 tablespoon red wine vinegar
2 tablespoons fresh basil, chopped	2 tablespoons fresh basil, chopped
1 teaspoon garlic, minced	1 teaspoon garlic, minced
1/4 teaspoon chili powder	1/4 teaspoon chili powder

2 cups tomatoes, sliced

3 ounces skim-milk mozzarella cheese, shredded

1 cup strawberries

2 cups tomatoes, sliced

4 ounces skim-milk mozzarella cheese, shredded

1 apple

Place lettuce on a serving plate. In a medium bowl, combine chickpeas, parsley, oil, vinegar, basil, garlic, and chili powder. Alternate slices of tomato and shredded mozzarella on the lettuce bed. Pour chickpea dressing over tomatoes and serve. Eat fruit for dessert.

Late-Afternoon Zone Snack

DINNER
❯ Indian Shrimp with Apples and Yogurt

Ingredients for women

1 teaspoon olive oil

3 ounces small shrimp, shelled and deveined

1/8 teaspoon fresh gingerroot, minced

1/2 teaspoon garlic, minced

1 tablespoon cilantro

Dash hot pepper sauce

1/4 teaspoon turmeric

1/8 teaspoon ground coriander

1/8 teaspoon ground cumin

2 teaspoons cider vinegar

1/2 cup plain low-fat yogurt

1/2 Granny Smith apple, diced

Ingredients for men

1 1/3 teaspoons olive oil

4 1/2 ounces small shrimp, shelled and deveined

1/8 teaspoon fresh gingerroot, minced

1/2 teaspoon garlic, minced

1 tablespoon cilantro

Dash hot pepper sauce

1/4 teaspoon turmeric

1/8 teaspoon ground coriander

1/8 teaspoon ground cumin

2 teaspoons cider vinegar

1/2 cup plain low-fat yogurt

1 Granny Smith apple, diced

3/4 cup onion, minced	3/4 cup onion, minced
5 cups romaine lettuce	5 cups romaine lettuce

Heat the oil in a medium nonstick sauté pan. Add shrimp and spices. Cook one to two minutes. In a second nonstick sauté pan, heat cider vinegar, yogurt, apple, and onion. When heated through, add shrimp mixture. Stir to mix. Form a bed of romaine on a serving plate and top with shrimp mixture.

Late-Evening Zone Snack

Fish Oil Requirements: Take at least 2.5 grams of EPA and DHA sometime during the day. Take more according to the guidelines in chapter 9 if you have the complications associated with Toxic Fat Syndrome.

Day 6

BREAKFAST
> Spanish Omelet

Ingredients for women
2 tablespoons yellow onion, peeled
    and finely chopped*
2 tablespoons green pepper, cored,
    seeded, and roughly chopped*
4 large egg whites (or 1/2 cup egg
    substitute)
1 tablespoon low-fat milk, optional
1 teaspoon chili powder or to taste,
    optional
1 teaspoon olive oil

Ingredients for men
2 tablespoons yellow onion, peeled
    and finely chopped*
2 tablespoons green pepper, cored,
    seeded, and roughly chopped*
6 egg whites (or 3/4 cup egg
    substitute)
1 tablespoon low-fat milk, optional
1 teaspoon chili powder or to taste,
    optional
1 1/3 teaspoons olive oil

¹/₄ cup canned black beans, drained and rinsed	¹/₂ cup canned black beans, drained and rinsed
1 ounce low-fat Monterey Jack cheese, shredded	1 ounce low-fat Monterey Jack cheese, shredded
1 tablespoon salsa, optional	1 tablespoon salsa, optional
1 medium orange	1 medium orange

Lightly coat a large nonstick sauté pan with vegetable spray and heat over medium flame. Add onion and green pepper and sauté, stirring often, until tender. Meanwhile, beat egg whites with milk, if desired. Stir in chili powder. Heat olive oil in another large, nonstick pan over medium heat. Pour in the egg whites and cook until almost set, occasionally lifting edges so that uncooked portion flows underneath, two to three minutes. When eggs are set, place onions, green pepper, black beans, and cheese on top. Fold with a spatula and continue cooking until lightly browned, about one minute. Top with salsa. Serve with orange.

Note: No one wants to chop vegetables first thing in the morning. Buy bags of frozen onions and green peppers and pour out what you need. Return the rest to the freezer.

LUNCH
> Dilled Chicken Salad

Ingredients for women	*Ingredients for men*
1 teaspoon olive oil	1¹/₃ teaspoons olive oil
3 ounces chicken tenderloin	4 ounces chicken tenderloin
2 cups mushrooms, sliced	2 cups mushrooms, sliced
1¹/₂ cups onion, chopped	1¹/₂ cups onion, chopped
¹/₈ teaspoon Worcestershire sauce	¹/₈ teaspoon Worcestershire sauce

¹/4 teaspoon lemon herb seasoning

1 tablespoon cider vinegar

1 teaspoon dried dill weed

Salt and pepper to taste

$1/2$ cup Zoned Herb Dressing
(see below)

5 cups romaine lettuce, torn

$1/4$ teaspoon lemon herb seasoning

1 tablespoon cider vinegar

1 teaspoon dried dill weed

Salt and pepper to taste

$1/2$ cup Zoned Herb Dressing
(see below)

5 cups romaine lettuce, torn

$1/2$ pear (for dessert)

Heat oil in medium nonstick sauté pan. Add chicken, mushrooms, onion, Worcestershire sauce, lemon and herb seasoning, cider vinegar, dill, and salt and pepper. Sauté until cooked through. Drain off excess liquid. Stir in Zoned Herb Dressing and simmer three to five minutes. Place chicken mixture on top of lettuce and serve.

> Zoned Herb Dressing

Ingredients

$1^{1}/2$ cups onion, finely minced

$1/4$ cup canned chickpeas, finely
minced

8 teaspoons cornstarch

$1^{3}/4$ cups water

$1/4$ cup cider vinegar

2 tablespoons balsamic vinegar

$1/8$ teaspoon Worcestershire sauce

1 teaspoon dried tarragon

1 teaspoon dried oregano

1 teaspoon parsley flakes

2 teaspoons garlic, minced

1 teaspoon dried basil

$1/8$ teaspoon chili powder

$1/2$ teaspoon celery salt

1 teaspoon dried dill

Combine all ingredients in a small saucepan to form a thickened dressing. (Mix cornstarch with a little cold water to dissolve it before adding to saucepan.) Heat dressing to a simmer, constantly stirring until mixture thickens. Transfer dressing mixture to a storage container, let cool, and refrigerate.

Note: This dressing may be refrigerated for up to five days, or if you prefer, the dressing may be frozen and thawed for later use. (Although the dressing is freeze-thaw stable, after dressing has been frozen and thawed, it may need to be stirred to reincorporate the small amount of moisture that forms on the dressing during the freezing and thawing process.)

Each $1/2$ cup equals 1 block of carbohydrate.

Late-Afternoon Zone Snack

DINNER
> Fish with Sautéed Vegetables

Ingredients for women	*Ingredients for men*
4$1/2$ ounces white fish, such as cod	6 ounces white fish, such as cod
1 dash lemon and lime juice	1 dash lemon and lime juice
Salt and fresh ground pepper	Salt and fresh ground pepper
1 teaspoon olive oil	1$1/3$ teaspoons olive oil
2 cups mushrooms, sliced	2 cups mushrooms, sliced
$3/4$ cup onion, sliced	$3/4$ cup onion, sliced
$1/4$ cup corn kernels, frozen	$1/4$ cup corn kernels, frozen
1$1/2$ cups chopped tomatoes	1$1/2$ cups chopped tomatoes
Basil and oregano to taste	Basil and oregano to taste
Salt and pepper to taste	Salt and pepper to taste
	1 peach (for dessert)

Preheat oven to 375 degrees. Put fish in shallow pan with a little water, sprinkle with lemon and lime juices, and add salt and pepper to taste. Bake fish until it flakes easily and is opaque throughout. While fish is baking, heat oil in large skillet and stir-fry veggies and add seasonings. Make a "bed" of the veggies and serve the fish on top.

Late-Evening Zone Snack

Fish Oil Requirements: Take at least 2.5 grams of EPA and DHA sometime during the day. Take more according to the guidelines in chapter 9 if you have the complications associated with Toxic Fat Syndrome.

Day 7

BREAKFAST

> Breakfast Burrito

Ingredients for women	*Ingredients for men*
$^1/_2$ cup egg substitute	$^3/_4$ cup egg substitute
1 teaspoon olive oil	$1^1/_3$ teaspoons olive oil
1 ounce fat-free cheese	1 ounce fat-free cheese
1 corn tortilla	1 corn tortilla
1 orange	1 orange
	$^3/_4$ cup V8 juice

Lightly coat sauté pan with olive oil and place over medium heat. Pour eggs into pan, scramble, and cook until set. Remove from pan, cool slightly, and add cheese. Gently roll up egg mixture in tortilla. Have fruit on the side.

LUNCH
> Vegetable Stew

Ingredients for women

3 soy hot dogs, sliced (21 grams of protein)

1 cup celery, sliced

1 cup scallions, sliced

1 cup carrots, finely diced

1$\frac{1}{2}$ cups tomato, chopped

9 olives

2 cups mushrooms, sliced

2 teaspoons garlic, minced

3 cups beef stock

2 tablespoons cider vinegar

$\frac{1}{8}$ teaspoon Worcestershire sauce

$\frac{1}{8}$ teaspoon dried oregano

Salt and pepper to taste

Ingredients for men

4 soy hot dogs, sliced (28 grams of protein)

1 cup celery, sliced

1 cup scallions, sliced

1 cup carrots, finely diced

1$\frac{1}{2}$ cups tomato, chopped

12 olives

2 cups mushrooms, sliced

2 teaspoons garlic, minced

3 cups beef stock

2 tablespoons cider vinegar

$\frac{1}{8}$ teaspoon Worcestershire sauce

$\frac{1}{8}$ teaspoon dried oregano

Salt and pepper to taste

1 peach (for dessert)

Combine all ingredients in a large saucepan. Bring to a boil; then simmer for thirty-five to forty minutes, until all vegetables are tender. Place mixture in a serving dish and serve immediately.

Late-Afternoon Zone Snack

DINNER

> Spiced Ground Beef with Vegetables

Ingredients for women	Ingredients for men
4^1/$_2$ ounces lean ground beef (or turkey or lamb)	6 ounces lean ground beef (or turkey or lamb)
1 teaspoon cider vinegar	1 teaspoon cider vinegar
1 tablespoon cilantro	1 tablespoon cilantro
2 teaspoons fresh ginger, minced	2 teaspoons fresh ginger, minced
^{1}/$_4$ teaspoon cumin	^{1}/$_4$ teaspoon cumin
^{1}/$_4$ teaspoon coriander	^{1}/$_4$ teaspoon coriander
^{1}/$_8$ teaspoon black pepper	^{1}/$_8$ teaspoon black pepper
^{1}/$_2$ teaspoon celery salt	^{1}/$_2$ teaspoon celery salt
^{1}/$_8$ teaspoon cinnamon	^{1}/$_8$ teaspoon cinnamon
1 teaspoon olive oil	1^1/$_3$ teaspoons olive oil
^{1}/$_2$ cup scallions, finely chopped	^{1}/$_2$ cup scallions, finely chopped
^{3}/$_4$ cup red onions, cut in chunks	^{3}/$_4$ cup red onions, cut in chunks
^{1}/$_4$ cup chickpeas	^{1}/$_4$ cup chickpeas
1 cup tomatoes, diced	1 cup tomatoes, diced
1^1/$_2$ cups green beans, diced	1^1/$_2$ cups green beans, diced
^{1}/$_8$ teaspoon cinnamon	^{1}/$_8$ teaspoon cinnamon
	1 plum (for dessert)

In a small glass bowl, combine meat, vinegar, and spices. Cover and refrigerate for thirty minutes. Heat the oil in a medium nonstick sauté pan. Add meat mixture and vegetables. Cook, breaking up meat, until it is cooked through and vegetables are tender. Spoon onto plate and serve.

Late-Evening Zone Snack

Fish Oil Requirements: Take at least 2.5 grams of EPA and DHA sometime during the day. Take more according to the guidelines in chapter 9 if you have the complications associated with Toxic Fat Syndrome.

Zone Snacks

Zone snacks have a very important role in the Zone dietary plan. They're not just a fun diversion to break up the day. Rather, they serve as hormonal touch-ups, taking us through the times when we don't have a meal for more than four to five hours. The first Zone snack is eaten either between breakfast and lunch or between lunch and dinner, depending upon which is the longer time span. For instance, a person who gets up at 6 a.m. should eat breakfast by 7. If that person doesn't eat lunch until 1 or 2 p.m., then a Zone snack should be eaten between breakfast and lunch. On the other hand, a person who eats breakfast at 9 a.m. will have a shorter time span between breakfast and lunch and a longer one between lunch and dinner, which means the snack should be eaten in the afternoon. The second Zone snack is eaten about one hour before bedtime to prevent nocturnal hypoglycemia.

A Zone snack is really a mini-Zone meal. Each contains one block of protein, one block of carbohydrate, and one block of fat. The following list of snack ideas comes from various Zone books and www.drsears.com. The list also offers some new options for Zoneful snacking.

Zone snack sizes are the same for men and women.

> DEVILED EGGS WITH HUMMUS

2 hard-boiled eggs
1/4 cup hummus (contains fat)
Paprika, optional

Slice the eggs in half, discard yolks, and fill each egg white with half the hummus. Top with paprika to taste.

> BAKED APPLE

1/2 gala apple, cored but not peeled
1/4 cup cottage cheese or 1 ounce low-fat cheese
1/2 teaspoon almond butter

Place apple half cut-side-up in baking dish and top with butter and a light sprinkle of cinnamon or nutmeg if desired. Bake in a 350-degree oven for about half an hour or until tender. Eat cheese on the side.

> LOW-FAT COTTAGE CHEESE AND FRUIT

1/4 cup low-fat cottage cheese
1/3 cup light fruit cocktail or 1/2 cup blueberries or
    1/2 chopped apple or 1/3 cup applesauce or 1 block of
    your favorite Zone-favorable fruit
1 macadamia nut or 3 almonds

> WANNA BE GREEK SALAD

1/2 cup green grapes
1 ounce Feta cheese

Cut the grapes in halves or thirds and put into bowl. Then mix the Feta cheese (either crumbled or cut into small pieces) with the grapes.

(This snack is popular with kids.)

> BERRY SMOOTHIE

7 grams protein powder

1 cup frozen raspberries, thawed

1 teaspoon slivered almonds

Blend the ingredients in a blender until smooth.

> TOMATO AND LOW-FAT MOZZARELLA SALAD

2 tomatoes, diced or sliced

1/3 teaspoon extra-virgin olive oil

Balsamic vinegar to taste

1 clove of garlic, minced

1 ounce skim mozzarella cheese

1 teaspoon chopped fresh basil leaves

Place tomatoes on a plate. In a small bowl, whisk together the olive oil, vinegar, and garlic. Pour the dressing over the tomatoes. Top with the cheese and basil.

> TUNA WITH HUMMUS

1 ounce canned tuna fish packed in water

1/4 cup hummus

Drain the tuna fish. Mix with the hummus.

› COTTAGE CHEESE AND SALSA

$1/4$ cup low-fat cottage cheese
$1/2$ cup salsa
1 tablespoon guacamole

Mix the ingredients together.

› WALDORF SALAD

1 cup celery, sliced
$1/4$ apple, diced
1 teaspoon light mayonnaise
1 pecan, crushed
1 ounce part-skim or "soft" cheese on the side

Put the celery and apple in a bowl. Mix in the light mayonnaise. Sprinkle the pecan pieces on top.

› LOW-FAT YOGURT AND NUTS

$1/2$ cup plain low-fat yogurt
1 teaspoon slivered almonds or 1 macadamia nut

› SPINACH SALAD

Spinach (side-salad size)
2 hard-boiled egg whites, sliced
$1/3$ cup mandarin oranges, canned in water
$1/3$ teaspoon olive oil

Balsamic vinegar to taste

Place the spinach on a plate. Top with egg whites and oranges. Whisk together the olive oil and vinegar and pour over the salad.

> TUNA FISH AND BLACK BEANS

1 ounce tuna fish
1/4 cup black beans
1 teaspoon low-fat mayonnaise

Mix together.

> VEGGIES AND DIP

2 ounces firm tofu
1/3 teaspoon olive oil
Dry onion soup mix to taste
1 cup celery, sliced for dipping
1 green pepper, sliced for dipping

In a small bowl, blend the tofu, olive oil, and soup mix. Serve with veggies.

> TOMATO AND LOW-FAT COTTAGE CHEESE

1/4 cup low-fat cottage cheese
2 tomatoes, sliced
6 peanuts

❯ CHEF SALAD

1 ounce sliced turkey or ham
Lettuce (side-salad size)
$1/4$ cup kidney beans
$1/3$ teaspoon olive oil
Balsamic vinegar to taste

Place the lettuce on a plate. Add the turkey or ham and kidney beans and toss with the olive oil and vinegar.

(This snack is popular with kids.)

❯ TACO SALAD

$11/2$ ounces ground turkey
Cooking spray
Taco seasoning to taste
1 tablespoon salsa
Lettuce (side-salad size)
$1/4$ cup black beans
1 tablespoon guacamole

Spray cooking spray into a small, nonstick sauté pan. Over medium heat, cook the turkey and sprinkle with taco seasoning. Place the lettuce on a plate and top with the turkey, salsa, beans, and guacamole.

❯ HAM AND FRUIT

$11/2$ ounces deli ham
$1/2$ apple
1 macadamia nut

❯ APPLESAUCE AND LOW-FAT CHEESE

$1/3$ cup applesauce

1 teaspoon slivered almonds

1 ounce low-fat cheese

❯ BERRIES AND LOW-FAT CHEESE

$1/2$ cup blueberries or 1 cup strawberries

1 ounce low-fat mozzarella cheese

6 peanuts

(This snack is popular with kids.)

❯ CHEESE AND APPLE

1 ounce part-skim mozzarella string cheese

$1/2$ apple

$1/2$ teaspoon natural peanut butter to spread on the apple

❯ WINE AND CHEESE

4 ounces red or white wine

1 ounce cheese

You can create an infinite variety of your very own Zone-favorable snacks. Choose one protein, one carbohydrate, and one fat choice from the list below.

PROTEINS:

- ➤ $1/4$ cup low-fat cottage cheese
- ➤ 1 ounce part-skim or light mozzarella
- ➤ $2^1/2$ ounces part-skim or light ricotta cheese
- ➤ 1 ounce sliced meat (turkey, ham, chicken)
- ➤ 1 ounce tuna packed in water
- ➤ 1 string cheese
- ➤ $1^1/2$ ounces deli meat

CARBOHYDRATES:

- ➤ $1/2$ apple
- ➤ 3 apricots
- ➤ 1 kiwi
- ➤ 1 tangerine
- ➤ $1/3$ cup light fruit cocktail
- ➤ $1/2$ pear
- ➤ 1 cup strawberries
- ➤ $3/4$ cup blackberries
- ➤ $1/2$ orange
- ➤ $1/2$ cup grapes
- ➤ 8 cherries
- ➤ $1/2$ nectarine
- ➤ 1 peach
- ➤ 1 plum
- ➤ $1/2$ cup light canned peaches

➤ 1 cup raspberries

➤ $1/2$ cup blueberries

➤ $1/2$ grapefruit

FATS:

➤ 3 olives (green or black)

➤ 1 macadamia nut

➤ 1 tablespoon guacamole

➤ 1 tablespoon avocado

➤ 3 almonds

➤ 6 peanuts

➤ 2 pecan halves

➤ $1/2$ teaspoon almond butter

➤ 1 teaspoon natural peanut butter

Continuing Support

B Y NOW I HOPE YOU REALIZE THAT MY DIETARY RECOMMENDATIONS may be the most powerful "drug" for living a longer and better life by reversing Toxic Fat Syndrome. This program is not a short-term diet but a way of life to treat food as if it were a medicine to maintain wellness. In essence, you are going back to the beginning of modern medicine and Hippocrates who is quoted as saying, "Let food be your medicine, and let medicine be your food."

Although this is the twelfth book I have written on the Zone, the printed word can only take you so far. That's why I have a staff of individuals trained to help you with every practical step of Zone living as well as to work with you as coaches to get you back to a state of wellness. My call center can be reached at 1-800-404-8171, or you can go to www.zonediet.com where you will find hundreds of Zone recipes, helpful hints, customized information, multiple discussion forums, and a wide variety of unique dietary products that make your entry into the Zone incredibly easy.

If you want more in-depth detail on the science of the Zone, then I suggest you go to www.drsears.com for up-to-the-minute information on the latest developments in this rapidly evolving field.

Blood Testing for Silent Inflammation

I BELIEVE THE MOST IMPORTANT BLOOD TEST YOU CAN EVER TAKE IS your fatty acid profile to determine the existence and extent of Toxic Fat Syndrome. This test will give you the arachidonic acid (AA)/eicosapentaenoic acid (EPA) and arachidonic acid (AA)/dihomo-gamma-linolenic acid (DGLA) ratios that are the markers for silent inflammation and cellular rejuvenation potential.

Ideally, you want the AA/EPA ratio to be less than 3 but not less than 1.5. Once this ratio is greater than 10, you can no longer be considered well. If the AA/EPA ratio exceeds 15, then you have high levels of silent inflammation in the blood (Toxic Fat Syndrome) that need immediate dietary attention.

Unfortunately, as important as this fatty acid profile test is, your physician has probably never heard of it, and it is not part of an annual physical. The reason is that the large clinical testing companies don't do this type of test, although it has been used in many research studies.

This is why I have spent a lot of effort developing a simple-to-use and inexpensive test using the newest analytical technology that requires only a finger prick to get enough blood to be placed on a piece of filter paper that has been impregnated with antioxidants to protect the fatty acids from oxidation. The dried blood spot on the filter paper is sent to my laboratory, and you get the results in five to ten working days. If you go to www.drsears.com or call Zone Labs at 800-404-8171, you will find the information on how to obtain this test.

There are other laboratories that do such fatty acid testing using larger amounts of blood that will require a physician's prescription. These include:

Nutrasource Diagnostics	519-824-4120 (Canada)
Kennedy Krieger Institute	443-923-2760
Metametrix Clinical Laboratory, Inc.	770-446-5483
Life Labs, Inc.	416-675-3637 (Canada)
Great Plains Laboratory, Inc.	913-341-8949
Carbon Based Corporation	775-851-3337
OmegaMetrix	816-931-0797

Hormones: The Keys to Your Biological Internet

UNTIL RECENTLY, WE THOUGHT OF HORMONES MAINLY IN TERMS of how wild they become during puberty. Now articles in every magazine refer to hormonal replacement with estrogen, testosterone, or growth hormone as the new elixirs of youth for an aging population.

While some hormones, such as estrogen, testosterone, and growth hormone, do decrease with age, others—such as insulin and pro-inflammatory eicosanoids—increase with age. It is these hormones that increase with age that can be rapidly modified by the Zone Diet. Ultimately by controlling both insulin and eicosanoids, you will achieve the fountain of youth (improved wellness) by reversing Toxic Fat Syndrome.

So what exactly is a hormone? The word *hormone* is derived from the Greek root meaning "impelling, exciting, or setting into motion." Hormones are exciting because they are hundreds of times more powerful than any drug. This is because they orchestrate complex cellular responses rather than affect a single enzyme.

A hormone can be considered to be any biochemical agent that can transmit information by calling a cell to action. Essentially, they are information messengers, just as electrons are mediators of information flow on the Internet. Likewise, hormones play the same role in your body, but they are far more complex in their interactions, allowing a greater texture and sophistication of information to be communicated.

Your Biological Internet

The key to understanding the Zone lies in knowing how hormones communicate to maintain equilibrium within your body. This is why I use the term "Biological Internet" to describe that interaction.

We marvel at the technological brilliance that made the Internet possible, yet within our bodies is a Biological Internet that is vastly more complex. Some 100 trillion cells need to maintain constant communication with one another. When your Biological Internet is working well, you're in a state of wellness. On the other hand, when it produces garbled information, you're heading toward chronic disease. The way to move from a chronic disease state to a state of improved wellness is to simultaneously reduce silent inflammation and increase your internal anti-inflammatory responses, both of which are controlled by eicosanoids. This is why eicosanoid control is at the core of your Biological Internet.

Subclasses of Hormones

Within your Biological Internet is a considerable subdivision of tasks, giving rise to three distinct classes of hormones called endocrine, paracrine, and autocrine. The differences between these types of hormones can be best illustrated by an analogy to your telephone.

Consider *endocrine* hormones to be like the microwave towers that send your telephone conversation into the air when you speak. Once the telephone signal is transmitted, it hopes to find the eventual location to which it is being directed. Likewise, endocrine hormones are sent from a secreting gland into the bloodstream with the eventual aim of finding the right cell (out of some 100 trillion cells) to communicate its message. Just like the telephone conversation relies upon the receiving microwave tower, a hormone needs to lock on to the right cell. That is done by binding to specific receptors on the cell surface. The hormone attaches onto the cell receptor like a spacecraft docking onto a space station.

Unlike endocrine hormones, *paracrine* hormones don't travel in the bloodstream. They are cell-to-cell regulators that have very defined routes to determine how far they can travel. In this respect, paracrine hormones are more like the physical telephone wires that come directly into your house after the signal is received by the microwave tower. Paracrine hormones don't need a supporting system like a bloodstream to carry them. All they need is either a nerve junction or very short pathway from the secreting cell to the target cell. Neurotransmitters, such as serotonin and dopamine, are examples of paracrine hormones. Paracrine hormones also work by binding to specific receptors.

The *autocrine* hormones are a type of molecular scout. These hormones are sent from a cell to test out the immediate environment and report back to that cell about what lies just outside its perimeter. These hormones also use receptors to report that information back to the cell. Taking our telephone analogy one step further, autocrine hormones are similar to the receiver of your phone. No matter how good the microwave towers (endocrine hormones) might be or the fidelity of the information transmitted via the telephone wires (paracrine hormones) to your home, unless the receiver (autocrine hormones) works properly, you are not going to have a telephone conversation. The most important autocrine hormones are the eicosanoids.

Transmitting Information into the Cell

Hormones still have to get the individual cell to respond to their signals. This is the job of second messengers and nuclear transcription factors.

Second Messengers

Second messengers are the key to the ability of a hormone to call a cell to action. The first step for most hormones, such as insulin, is to dock with its receptor on the cell surface. This hormone receptor, which spans the membrane of the cell, undergoes a structural change that is transmitted to a particular enzyme through different membrane-bound proteins known as G proteins. Once activated by a hormone outside the cell, a second messenger is made inside the cell, and this completes the original message. There are two primary second messengers for all cells. In essence, much of the complexity of hormonal interaction becomes reduced to a biochemical traffic signal with either a green or a red light.

Among the most important of these molecular traffic lights is cyclic AMP. (The 1971 Nobel Prize in Medicine was awarded for the discovery of this molecule.) Cyclic AMP can be considered the green light for the cell, and it starts a new cascade of information transmission (via protein kinase A) that tells the cell what to do. Good eicosanoids interact with receptors that produce this second messenger.

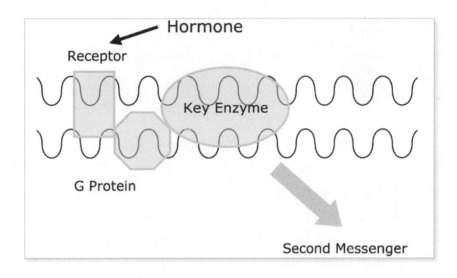

The other major second messenger system is called the inositol triphosphate/diacylglycerol (IP_3/DAG) pathway. This is equivalent to a red light in the cell because it usually has the opposite physiological action of cyclic AMP as it activates a different casacade via protein kinase C. Both insulin and pro-inflammatory eicosanoids use this pathway. Think of these second messengers as the internal traffic signals in each of your 100 trillion cells as shown in the following chart.

Hormonal Action Is Based on the Balance of Second Messengers

cAMP $\longrightarrow$ PKA

IP$_3$ /DAG $\longrightarrow$ PKC

If the balance of green and red lights is working smoothly, the result is wellness. If the traffic signals are out of balance, chronic disease results. In the final analysis, the great complexity of your Biological Internet comes down to maintaining the appropriate balance of green and red lights in each of the trillions of cells throughout your body so that information traffic flows efficiently.

Nuclear Transcription Factors

Another group of intracellular hormone receptors is called nuclear transcription factors. Once these factors are activated, they go directly into the nucleus of the cell to stimulate your genes to increase the production of new proteins. The two most important of these are nuclear factor-kappaB (NF-kappaB) and peroxisome proliferator activated receptors (PPAR).

NF-kappaB controls the inducible inflammatory actions of the cell.

Once this transcription factor is activated, it causes the gene expression of a wide variety of inflammatory enzymes (COX-2) and cytokines (TNF alpha and IL-6) that amplify the original inflammatory signal.

PPAR is really a family of transcription factors, including PPAR-alpha and PPAR-gamma. If PPAR-alpha is activated, it causes genes to produce a variety of enzymes that oxidize fat. If PPAR-gamma is activated, it reduces insulin resistance by increasing the formation of new, healthy fat cells (good fat) as well as increasing the formation of unique anti-inflammatory eicosanoids.

Fatty acids released into the interior of the cell from its membrane and the eicosanoids derived from those released fatty acids can also act as second messengers by either activating or inhibiting these same nuclear transcription factors.

Hormones and Appetite Regulation

The reason that you gain weight is because your hormones are out of balance. The way to lose weight is to bring your hormones back into balance. In other words, you have to maintain them in a zone that is not too high but not too low.

Although I have previously discussed the importance of several hormones that are key in the control of hunger and satiety, this appendix becomes an ideal place to give you a little more detail on the complexity of this intricate control system. Ultimately, much of the action takes place at the base of the hypothalamus in an area known as the arcuate nucleus. Within this location are both appetite-stimulating and appetite-suppressing neurons. If the satiety neurons are stimulated, then the hormone melanocortin is secreted. On the other hand, if the hunger neurons are stimulated, then there is the release of neuropeptide

Y (NPY), the hormone that stimulates hunger as well as agouri-related peptide (known as AGRP) that inhibits the satiety action of melanocortin. Depending upon which set of neurons in the arcuate nucleus is activated, an integrated signal is sent to the paraventricular nucleus (PVN) of the hypothalamus, which ultimately determines whether you should eat or not.

The activation of the satiety and hunger neurons is affected by a wide variety of hormones sending in information from diverse locations throughout the body. Both leptin and insulin can inhibit the actions of the stimulation of the hunger neurons, thus increasing satiety. (This is why if you push insulin levels too low, you get hungry again.) Thus, overcoming insulin resistance and leptin resistance (both mediated by silent inflammation) in the central nervous system is necessary if you want to increase satiety. Fortunately, this can be accomplished by using the combination of the Zone Diet and high-dose fish oil.

Although the digestive system is a great distance from the brain, it, too, can play a significant role in hunger and satiety. The hormone ghrelin, secreted from the stomach, is activated by the lack of food. Its release from the stomach goes directly to the brain to activate the hunger neurons, thus releasing both NPY and AGRP, which makes you hungry. However, another hormone, PYY (stimulated by dietary protein), is secreted from the ileum, and the colon can inhibit the action of ghrelin. This provides a nice "on-off" system to signal to the brain from different parts of the digestive system as to when to start and stop eating. As I mentioned earlier, obese patients have reduced levels of PYY, so they have a reduced "off" switch when it comes to appetite control. Among one of the most widely studied gut hormones is cholecystokinin (CCK). CCK is released from the duodenum in response to fats and protein. This not only causes the release of bile from the gallbladder to help emulsify fat for absorption but also sends a satiety signal to the brain. Unfortunately, the satiety actions of CCK are very short-lived, having a half life measured in minutes, but it does appear that CCK helps stimulate PYY release, which has a greater long-term effect on satiety.

One of the reasons that gastric bypass surgery appears to be successful is because after the surgery there is a much greater PYY response to food, thus helping to increase satiety. (Obviously, there are better ways to increase release of PYY, such as following the Zone Diet rather than cutting out healthy tissue.)

Besides these above-mentioned gut hormones that can directly affect the neurons in the arcuate nucleus, there are other gut hormones (such as GLP-1 and oxyntomodulin) also involved in this intricate hormonal regulation of appetite. It appears that the digestive system has a wide range of hormonal sensors, from the stomach all the way down to the colon, that constantly transmit information to the brain about when to eat and, more importantly, when to stop eating.

The last major players in the brain that can override this intricate balance of external endocrine hormones on the satiety and hunger neurons in the arcuate nucleus are the endocannabinoids, derived from increased levels of toxic fat (AA) in the brain. These hunger-inducing hormones can override the delicate hormonal balance in the arcuate nucleus to increase appetite. The best way to reduce elevated endocannabinoid levels is to ensure that you are following the Zone Diet (to reduce the formation of AA) and consuming adequate levels of EPA to dilute excess AA in the brain.

Paracrine hormones, such as dopamine and serotonin, in the brain also have a role to play in the regulation of appetite. One of the oldest prescription drugs for weight loss is phentermine, which causes the release of dopamine, which in turn gives rise to appetite suppression.

Phentermine has limited effectiveness because it can also cause an increase in blood pressure, dry mouth, insomnia, constipation, and nervousness. Thus, it is usually limited to only twelve weeks of use. An interesting side note is when you combine phentermine with fenfluramine (a drug that maintains a high level of serotonin by simultaneously preventing its uptake, like other antidepressant drugs, as well as enhancing its release) to reduce the nervous, edgy feeling induced by phentermine alone, you get a lot of appetite suppression coupled with a happier disposition. This combination of drugs was known as Fen-Phen. Since the side effects of phentermine were eliminated, millions of people (and their physicians) thought they could keep taking this drug combination for a long time. Unfortunately, the combination of these two drugs had a dual problem of causing primary pulmonary hypertension (that can be corrected only by both a heart transplant and a lung transplant) and damage to heart valves by the overstimulation of serotonin release. This is a pretty dangerous way to lose weight. I know since I was the obesity expert in the class action suit against the manufacturer of fenfluramine. Fortunately, the judge agreed with me and the other experts that fenfluramine was simply a very dangerous drug. As a result, it cost the maker of fenfluramine close to $19 billion to settle all the lawsuits.

There is one other endocrine hormone derived from the adipose tissue that can affect fat accumulation without directly affecting the hunger and satiety neurons in the brain. This is the hormone adiponectin, which is secreted from the fat cells to reduce insulin resistance. One of the best ways to increase adiponectin levels is the increased consumption of fish oil, which appears to increase its production via the stimulation of the PPAR-gamma gene transcription factor.

I think you can begin to understand from this very short description of the role of hormones on appetite regulation that weight gain may have very little to do with lack of willpower or catchy marketing campaigns by the food giants, but it is primarily caused by imbalances in your hormones that can be modulated by an anti-inflammatory diet, like the Zone Diet, coupled with high-dose fish oil.

Summary

Each of your 100 trillion cells is controlled by hormonal signals that switch on or switch off complex internal molecular functions on a second-by-second basis. Your wellness (as well as your hunger) depends upon keeping these hormones in balance. If they are out of balance, obesity and chronic disease accelerate. Maintaining yourself in the Zone gives you that hormonal control.

Eicosanoids: Hormones of Mystery

THE WORD *EICOSANOID* EVEN SOUNDS LIKE IT CAME FROM SCIENCE fiction. After all, these hormones are strange, mysterious, and almost mystical. Yet as important as eicosanoids are, few physicians know anything about them, even though these hormones control the levels of silent inflammation as well as regulate your body's internal cellular rejuvenation capacity.

Eicosanoids can be considered "super-hormones" because they control directly or indirectly the hormonal actions of virtually every other hormone. You don't have a unique eicosanoid gland: every one of your 100 trillion cells can make eicosanoids. Our knowledge of eicosanoids started with the discovery of essential fatty acids in 1929. It was found that if all the fats in the diet were removed, the test animals would soon die. Adding back certain essential fats (then called vitamin F) allowed the fat-deprived test animals to live. Eventually as technologies advanced, researchers realized that essential fats were composed of both omega-6 and omega-3 fatty acids, and both had to be obtained in the diet because the body could not synthesize them. However, not all essential fatty acids can be made into eicosanoids. Only those essential fatty acids that are twenty carbon atoms in length—arachidonic acid (AA), dihomo-gamma-linolenic acid (DGLA), and eicosapentaenoic acid (EPA)—can be made into eicosanoids. That is why the word *eicosanoids* is derived from the Greek word for "twenty," which is *eicosa*.

Ulf von Euler discovered the first eicosanoids in 1935. These were isolated from the prostate gland (an exceptionally rich source of eicosanoids), and were called prostaglandins (a small subset of the much larger family of eicosanoids). It was thought at that time that all hormones had to originate from a discrete gland, so it made perfect sense to name this new hormone a *prostaglandin*. Today we know that every living cell in the body can make eicosanoids, and that there is no discrete organ or gland that is the center of eicosanoid synthesis.

To date, biochemists have identified more than one hundred eicosanoids and are finding more each year. The breakthrough in eicosanoid research occurred in 1971 when John R. Vane finally discovered how aspirin (the wonder drug of the twentieth century) worked: it changed the levels of eicosanoids. Vane and his colleagues, Bengt Samuelsson and Sune Bergström, received the 1982 Nobel Prize in Medicine for their discoveries of the role eicosanoids play in human disease.

Why are eicosanoids so unknown if they are so important? First, they are made, act, and self-destruct within seconds, which makes them very hard to study. Second, they don't circulate in the bloodstream, so trying to sample them is extremely difficult. Finally, they work at incredibly low concentrations, making it almost impossible to detect them. Despite these barriers, more than one hundred thousand articles on eicosanoids have been published in peer-reviewed journals. At least the basic research community is interested in eicosanoids, even if your doctor never learned about them in medical school.

Eicosanoids encompass a wide array of hormones, many of which endocrinologists have never heard of. The different classes of eicosanoids include:

Endocannabinoids
Epi-lipoxins
Hydroxylated fatty acids
Leukotrienes
Lipoxins
Prostaglandins
Resolvins
Thromboxanes

Just about every physician has heard of prostaglandins. However, prostaglandins are only a small subgroup of the eicosanoid family. Some of the other subgroups were only discovered recently. For example, aspirin-triggered epi-lipoxins and resolvins are eicosanoids that give rise to powerful anti-inflammatory properties and were discovered only a few years ago. In fact, it was discovered in 2006 that virtually any drug that binds to the nuclear transcription factor PPAR-gamma will also induce production of anti-inflammatory epi-lipoxins.

Biological response modifiers are molecules that orchestrate extensive changes in the cell. Eicosanoids represent probably the most powerful of these modifiers and play a central role in our physiology. The cell surface has a variety of eicosanoid receptors, and depending on which eicosanoid interacts with a specific receptor, a second messenger is synthesized by the cell. Sometimes a second messenger such as cyclic AMP is generated, and sometimes a totally different second messenger, such as the IP_3/DAG system, is generated. If one of these second messengers increases, then the other will decrease.

Good and Bad Eicosanoids

The second messenger that a particular eicosanoid produces becomes the molecular definition of a good or bad eicosanoid. A good eicosanoid will increase the levels of cyclic AMP in a cell, while a bad eicosanoid will decrease the levels of cyclic AMP through the elevation of the levels of the IP_3/DAG second messengers. The following table lists the types of good and bad eicosanoids and the receptors with which they interact.

Receptors for Good and Bad Eicosanoids		
Good Eicosanoids		
	Receptor	Effect on Cyclic AMP
PGE_1	EP2, EP4	increase
PGI_2	IP	increase
PGD_2	DP	increase

Receptors for Good and Bad Eicosanoids		
Bad Eicosanoids		
	Receptor	Effect on Cyclic AMP
TXA_2	TP	decrease
PGE_2	EP1, EP3	decrease
$PGF_{2\alpha}$	FP	decrease
LTB_4	BLT	decrease
LTC_4	Cys-LTi	decrease
LTD_4, LTE_4	CysLT2	decrease

Once an eicosanoid interacts with its unique receptor, a second messenger is synthesized inside the target cell. If a good eicosanoid interacts with the right receptor, then cyclic AMP is the second messenger formed. On the other hand, if a bad eicosanoid interacts with its receptor, then cyclic AMP levels are decreased. Further complicating this is that some eicosanoids, such as PGA and PGJ, are cyclopentenone eicosanoids. These eicosanoids don't have cell receptors on the surface but can directly activate nuclear transcription factors inside the cell. These then interact directly with the cell's nucleus via nuclear transcription factors (like the PPAR) to affect cellular growth and differentiation.

Because there is no discrete eicosanoid gland, there is no central site that turns eicosanoid action "on" or "off." Instead, our body produces different types of eicosanoids that have diametrically opposed physiological actions. A balance of these opposing physiological actions of different eicosanoids is required to maintain a balance of opposing biological actions. These differences in biological actions are the foundation for the eicosanoid "axis." This means the body must constantly play a balancing game to maintain wellness. This eicosanoid axis is composed of good eicosanoids on one side and bad eicosanoids on the other. Obviously, there is no such thing as an absolutely good eicosanoid or an absolutely bad eicosanoid. It's just when you start making more bad eicosanoids and fewer good eicosanoids that bad things begin to happen.

Virtually all chronic diseases can be viewed as a consequence of a continuing imbalance of good and bad eicosanoids. This is the insight I gained from the 1982 Nobel Prize in Medicine. It also became apparent to me that the appropriate balance of eicosanoids could be used to provide the molecular definition of wellness. In essence, the more the balance of eicosanoids is tilted toward bad eicosanoids, the more likely you are to develop chronic disease. Conversely, the more the balance is tilted toward good eicosanoids, the greater the chance that you'll achieve wellness and longevity. The AA/DGLA ratio will indicate where you stand in terms of the body's ability to increase cellular rejuvenation (anti-aging). On the other hand, the AA/EPA ratio will tell you the extent of silent inflammation in the body. That is why you want both ratios to be optimized.

How Eicosanoids Are Synthesized

Because eicosanoids are produced in every cell—not one specific gland—it's as if you have 100 trillion separate eicosanoid glands capable of making these exceptionally powerful hormones. Unlike the endocrine hormones, which are under control of the hypothalamus and the pituitary gland, there is no such central control on eicosanoids. Rather than responding to some master signal, each cell responds to changes in its immediate environment. The only fatty acids that can be synthesized into eicosanoids are AA, DGLA, and EPA. These fatty acids are stored as phospholipids, which are integral components of every cell membrane. The first step in generating a cellular response is the actual release of one of these twenty carbon chain essential fatty acids from the phospholipids in the cell membrane. The enzyme responsible for the release of the essential fatty acid is called phospholipase A_2.

Because no hormonal feedback loop exists to stop the production of eicosanoids, the only way to inhibit their release from the membrane is by the production of corticosteroids (such as cortisol) from the adrenal gland. This causes the synthesis of a protein (lipocortin) that inhibits the action of phospholipase A_2. By inhibiting this enzyme, which releases essential fatty acids from the cell membranes, you choke off the supply of a substrate required for all eicosanoid synthesis. Obviously, if you are overproducing cortisol (especially during stress), you will bring all eicosanoid synthesis (good and bad) to a grinding halt. This can cause your immune system to begin to shut down.

Upstream Versus Downstream Pharmacology

It's not that drug companies are ignorant of eicosanoids. They have developed a vast array of anti-inflammatory drugs to inhibit the enzymes that synthesize eicosanoids. Unfortunately, these anti-inflammatory drugs are like dumb bombs. They knock out the production of both good and bad eicosanoids. This was the problem with Vioxx and the cause of the side effects with long-term use of corticosteroids.

In pharmacology, the use of drugs to inhibit the production of another key biochemical is known as "going downstream." However, a far more elegant approach is to "go upstream" by simply changing the balance of the precursors of eicosanoids so you are more likely to make a good eicosanoid and less likely to make a bad eicosanoid. This is what makes the Zone Diet such a powerful program because it can choke off the production of arachidonic acid. The Zone Diet can accomplish what no drug can in manipulating the balance of the most powerful hormones in the body. To understand how that is possible, you have to understand the impact of the diet on the synthesis of essential fatty acids (AA, DGLA, and EPA) that drive eicosanoid synthesis.

Synthesis of Essential Fatty Acids

All eicosanoids ultimately are produced from essential fatty acids that the body cannot make, and therefore must be part of the diet. These essential fatty acids are classified as either omega-3 or omega-6, depending upon the position of their double bonds. Only plants and algae have the capacity to insert such double bonds using specific delta-12- or delta-15-desaturase enzymes that mammals cannot make. This is why the dietary inclusion of these fatty acids is essential for life. However, man has the ability to insert other double bonds into these fatty acids at other positions.

Typical omega-3 and omega-6 essential fatty acids in the diet are only eighteen carbons long and must be further elongated to twenty-carbon fatty acids by the body before eicosanoids can be made. Remember, all eicosanoids have come from essential fatty acids that are twenty carbon atoms in length. It is not just the number of carbon atoms that count, but also their configuration. Eicosanoid precursors must have a certain spatial configuration with at least three conjugated double bonds in order to be converted into an eicosanoid.

The differences between the two classes of essential fatty acids,

261

omega-6 and omega-3, are based on the position of the double bonds within the fatty acid molecule. This is important because it is the positioning of these double bonds that dictates their three-dimensional structure in space that ultimately determines how they interact with their appropriate receptors. Although the synthesis of longer chain-essential fatty acids uses many of the same enzymes, their metabolic pathways are quite different. Because the metabolism of long-chain omega-3 fatty acids is more complex, let's start with the simpler pathway to make omega-6 fatty acids.

Omega-6 Fatty Acids

There are two key metabolic steps in this process that determine the amounts of actual eicosanoid building blocks that can be made, known in biochemistry as "rate-limiting steps." The first rate-limiting step is controlled by the enzyme delta-6-desaturase. This enzyme inserts a necessary third double bond in the essential fatty acid in just the right

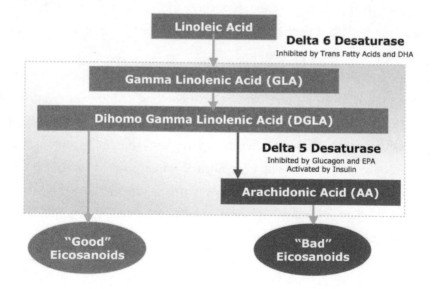

position to begin bending inward and forms gamma-linolenic acid (GLA) from linoleic acid as shown in the figure on the opposite page.

Once this new double bond has been inserted into a short-chain essential fatty acid to form GLA, then very small amounts of these newly formed essential fatty acids can profoundly affect eicosanoid balance in your body.

However, many factors can decrease the activity of delta-6-desaturase enzyme. The most important factor is age itself. There are two times during your life that this enzyme is relatively inactive. The first is at birth. For the first six months of life, the activity of this key enzyme in the newborn is relatively low. But this is also the time in which maximum amounts of long-chain essential fatty acids are required by the child as the brain is growing at the fastest possible rate, and these long-chain essential fatty acids are the key structural building blocks for the brain. The solution to this problem: breast milk. Breast milk is very rich in GLA and other long-chain essential fatty acids such as EPA and DHA (docosahexacnoic acid). By supplying these essential fatty acids through the diet, this early inactivity of the delta-6-desaturase enzyme is overcome.

The second time in your life during which the activity of this enzyme begins to decrease is after the age of thirty. Eicosanoids are critical for successful reproduction. The primary child-bearing years for women are between the ages of eighteen and thirty. Therefore, the activity of a key enzyme needed to make the precursors of eicosanoids required for fertility begins to diminish after the age of thirty.

The delta-6-desaturase enzyme can also be inhibited by viral infection. The only known antiviral agents are good eicosanoids, such as PGA_1, because of their ability to increase cyclic AMP levels that keep viral replication under control. Therefore, the number-one goal of the virus is to inhibit the formation of this type of eicosanoid. This is exactly what many viruses do by inhibiting the delta-6-desaturase enzyme. By doing so, the virus has devised an incredibly clever way to circumvent the body's primary antiviral defense (PGA_1).

The final factor that can decrease the activity of delta-6-desaturase is the presence of two types of fatty acids in your diet: trans fats and omega-3 fats. Trans fatty acids don't exist naturally but are easily produced by food manufacturers. They are omega-6 fatty acids that have been chemically transformed by a commercial process known as hydrogenation into a new spatial configuration that is more stable to prevent oxidation. The increased stability of these fatty acids makes them ideal for extending the shelf life of processed foods, but also their change in molecular configuration makes them strong inhibitors of the delta-6-desaturase enzyme. Trans fatty acids occupy the active site of the delta-6-desaturase enzyme, thus preventing the formation of the activated essential fatty acids required for eicosanoid synthesis. In essence, trans fatty acids can be viewed as anti-essential fatty acids because of their inhibition of eicosanoid synthesis. This may be why they are strongly implicated in the development of heart disease. How do you know if a food product you're consuming contains trans fatty acids? Look for the phrase "partially hydrogenated vegetable oil" on the label. If it is there, the food contains trans fatty acids.

Surprisingly, omega-3 fatty acids can also inhibit this same enzyme, with DHA having the greatest impact. This is one of the problems of trying to use only fish oil to modulate eicosanoid synthesis. The EPA in fish oil can help reduce silent inflammation, but the DHA reduces the production of GLA required to make good eicosanoids.

The metabolic progression of an omega-6 fatty acid toward becoming an eicosanoid building block is still far from over after passing this first hurdle of making GLA. Once GLA is formed, it is rapidly elongated into dihomo-gamma-linolenic acid (DGLA), which is the precursor to many of the good eicosanoids. However, DGLA is also the substrate for the other rate-limiting enzyme in the essential fatty acid cascade: delta-5-desaturase. The activity of the delta-5-desaturase enzyme ultimately controls the balance of good and bad eicosanoids. If your goal is to treat chronic disease and promote wellness, you want to modulate the activity of this enzyme. Decrease the activity of delta-5-desaturase, and you make more of the building blocks (DGLA) for good eicosanoids. Increase the activity of the same enzyme, and you produce more building blocks (AA) for bad eicosanoids. The activity of this key enzyme is ultimately controlled by your diet because of the stimulatory impact of insulin.

As delta-5-desaturase activity increases, DGLA goes down and AA goes up. This can be seen by the increasing AA/DGLA ratio in the blood. Ultimately, the balance between DGLA and AA in every one of your 100 trillion cells determines which types of eicosanoids you will produce. You need some AA to produce some bad eicosanoids, but with excess production of AA, the balance of eicosanoids will shift toward accelerated development of chronic disease.

Many of these eicosanoids (especially PGE_2 and LTB_4), derived from arachidonic acid, promote inflammation. In addition, these inflammatory eicosanoids can also promote the release of other pro-inflammatory mediators by activating NF-kappaB. Once activated, NF-kappaB goes directly to the nucleus, activating the synthesis of more inflammatory mediators that amplify the intensity of immunological attack.

While there is a bewildering complexity of eicosanoids from AA, a very limited number of eicosanoids can be synthesized from DGLA.

The primary eicosanoid derived from DGLA is PGE_1, one of the most highly studied good eicosanoids and a very powerful vasodilator and inhibitor of platelet aggregation. It also reduces the secretion of insulin and increases the synthesis of a wide variety of hormones that normally decrease during the aging process. PGE_1 can achieve these diverse functions because it causes an increase in cyclic AMP production. PGA_1 is the most powerful suppressor of viral replication, especially HIV transcription, as well as inhibiting nuclear transcription factor NF-kappaB necessary for synthesis of a wide variety of pro-inflammatory cytokines. DGLA can also be converted into a powerful inhibitor that decreases leukotriene synthesis (such as LTB_4). You can see that having higher levels of DGLA compared to AA plays an important role in decreasing inflammation.

Omega-3 Fatty Acids

The synthesis of long-chain omega-3 fatty acids is much more complex than the omega-6 fatty acids.

The synthetic sequence of omega-3 fatty acids from alpha-linolenic acid to EPA formation is seemingly relatively straightforward, just like the synthesis of AA is from its short-chain precursor (linoleic acid). In fact, the same enzymes are used in both pathways. However, alpha-linolenic acid is another inhibitor of the delta-6-desaturase enzyme, just like DHA. This feedback inhibition makes the formation of EPA much more difficult than it should be. This is why studies comparing the dietary intake of ALA versus EPA have indicated that the efficiency of making EPA from ALA is extremely limited. Therefore, if you want to get the greatest benefit of EPA, it will have to come from consuming fish oil, not vegetable sources rich in ALA (such as flaxseed).

Omega-3 fatty acid synthesis gets even more complex as it goes through additional synthetic steps to make DHA, which is critical for brain function. EPA must be elongated and then converted again by the delta-6-desaturase enzyme to the precursor of DHA, which then must be shortened by perioxisomal enzymes into DHA. The result is that the synthesis of DHA from ALA is even more difficult than the synthesis of EPA (which isn't very good to begin with). Furthermore, because DHA used the delta-6-desaturase enzyme in its synthesis, its mere presence acts as a feedback inhibitor of the delta-6-desaturase enzyme that further reduces the flow of ALA to EPA and DHA. More ominously, the same inhibition of delta-6-desaturase by DHA also restricts the production of DGLA, thus reducing cellular rejuvenation potential.

The Role of Insulin

The most efficient way of decreasing AA formation is by reducing the dietary intake of omega-6 fatty acids found in vegetable oils coupled with a reduction of insulin levels using the Zone Diet. Under normal conditions, the synthesis of AA and EPA from their shorter-chain precursors (linoleic and alpha-linolenic acids respectively) is a slow process, controlled by two distinct rate-limiting enzymes (delta-6-desaturase and delta-5-desaturase). All bets are off when insulin levels increase, as this hormone is a powerful activator of both enzymes. As insulin levels rise (especially due to insulin resistance), the otherwise orderly synthesis of long-chain essential fatty acids gets accelerated and becomes controlled by the dietary ratio of omega-6 to omega-3 fatty acids. Because that ratio has been greatly increased due to the increased consumption of cheap vegetable oils rich in linoleic acid, the normal, healthy balance of AA/EPA becomes increased, leading to increased silent inflammation. Left untreated, this results in the acceleration of a wide number of chronic diseases that are a consequence of Toxic Fat Syndrome.

If your AA/EPA ratio is too high, then you have two dietary options. The first, and most effective, is to follow the Zone Diet and exclude as many omega-6 fatty acids as possible from your diet. This will reduce the total amount of AA in your body. The second option is to increase the intake of EPA in your diet. This will dilute out the excess AA in your body. Ideally, you should be doing both.

The Spillover Effect

Twenty-five years ago, I thought that simply controlling the ratio of AA to DGLA by adding the right amount of GLA to fish oil would be all that I needed to control eicosanoids. I described in chapter 9 the complexity of this approach. Although the use of additional inhibitors of delta-5-desaturase (such as toasted sesame oil concentrates) can help prevent the spillover of DGLA into AA, it is still a tricky process. This is why if you consider adding any GLA to your diet, you also want to be following the Zone Diet to reduce the levels of insulin that would otherwise activate the same delta-5-desaturase enzyme that produces AA. You will also need to take at least one hundred times more EPA compared to the levels of supplemented GLA not to have problems. The manipulation of the ratio of AA and DGLA in every cell in your body can be done, but it is tricky.

Everything You Ever Wanted to Know About Fish Oil But Were Afraid to Ask

ERE'S AN OBVIOUS QUESTION: WHY NOT SIMPLY CONSUME A lot of fish instead of taking fish oil supplements? The Japanese do, and they have low levels of Toxic Fat Syndrome and the greatest longevity in the world.

The problem is that all fish are contaminated. There is simply no place on the face of the earth where fish are not contaminated with either mercury (primarily from coal burning); persistent toxins that are no longer manufactured, such as PCBs and dioxins; and new toxins, such as flame retardants, that are not yet banned in the United States. All of these are found in fish, and the more fish you eat, the more of these persistent toxins you accumulate. This is why the blood levels of these toxins in the Japanese population are near the upper limits set by the World Health Organization.

The other problem is you have to consume significant amounts of fish to lower the levels of silent inflammation. Currently Americans consume about 125 milligrams per day of EPA (eicosapentaenoic acid) and DHA (docosahexaenoic acid). My clinical data indicate it requires the consumption of nearly twenty times that amount (about 2.5 grams of EPA and DHA per day) before you begin to significantly lower the levels of silent inflammation. That's a lot of fish. That's why I believe the only reasonable answer is the consumption of fish oils rich in EPA and DHA that are free of toxins. Fortunately, they do exist, but before I describe them, let me give you a little history on fish oil production.

The History of Fish Oil

Extracting fish oil is relatively straightforward. Simply boil the fish until the oil rises to the top of the vat, a process known as rendering. Unfortunately, this crude fish oil also represents the sewer of the sea, since fish are at the end of the food chain in the ocean, and anything in that food chain that contains fat-soluble toxins, such as PCBs, dioxins, and organic mercury compounds, will be concentrated in the rendered oil. The big problem is how to make crude fish oil suitable for human consumption.

The first recorded medical use of fish oil occurred in 1789 in England. When cod was brought back from America, the livers were left to ferment in tubs. After many days of fermentation, the oil would ooze out and could be collected. Disgusting as it was, this crude cod-liver oil was considered a miracle cure for arthritis. The big manufacturing "breakthrough" in cod-liver oil production occurred in 1854 with the boiling of the livers in an iron pot. The cod-liver oil was still disgusting.

Fast-forward to the end of the nineteenth century, when the first

Chinese immigrants brought sea snake oil to America. Sea snakes feed on fish, and as a consequence, the oil in their system is rich in EPA and DHA. The percentage of EPA and DHA in sea snake oil is approximately double that found in cod-liver oil, so at the end of the nineteenth century, sea snake oil was the most potent source of EPA and DHA known to medicine. Not surprisingly, it was touted as being a cure for everything (and it probably was because it was the best anti-inflammatory drug available at the time). It also tasted terrible (even worse than cod-liver oil). Thus, it became very easy for hucksters to put any foul-tasting substance in a bottle and try to sell it as "just as good as sea snake oil, but only cheaper." Hence, the term "snake oil salesman" became a common part of our language.

In the 1930s, consumption of a tablespoon of cod-liver oil became standard practice for every child because it was the best treatment for preventing rickets, as it is rich in vitamin D. Along with the vitamin D, these children were getting a good dose of EPA and DHA (about 2.5 grams per day).

Obviously, we've come a long way from letting cod-livers ferment to release their oil or selling sea snake oil. Yet even modern cod-liver oil is full of industrial contaminants, such as mercury, PCBs, and dioxins, and shark-liver oil is even worse. And it has the same foul taste that turned the stomachs of every child in America who took cod-liver oil two generations ago. So while it's true that one tablespoon of cod-liver oil would supply 2.5 grams of long-chain omega-3 fatty acids—what I consider a maintenance dose—it also supplies contaminants and a high dose of vitamin A, which is stored in the body's fat tissues and can possibly cause toxic effects, such as hair loss, or worse, if taken in high enough doses.

In the 1980s, fish oil manufacturing finally took a technological leap forward. Manufacturers began extracting the oil from the body, instead of the liver, of the fish. This solved the problem of potential vitamin A toxicity (because the liver contains all the vitamin A). These fish body oils, however, tasted just as bad as cod-liver oil, so consumers were still reluctant to try them. Manufacturers solved this problem by encapsulating the oil in soft gelatin capsules. The only problem was that the capsules often cost ten times the value of the fish oil inside them.

Although fish oil capsules solved the initial taste problem, they also created a new one—no one was taking enough EPA and DHA to get a therapeutic dose. For example, to get the same amount of EPA and DHA provided by a tablespoon of cod-liver oil required eight relatively large 1-gram capsules of fish body oil per day. To get the amount of EPA and DHA used in the Harvard Medical School study to treat bipolar depression, a person would have to take more than thirty 1-gram capsules per day. The one or two capsules a day that most of us are willing to take have little effect because the amount of long-chain omega-3 fatty acids found at that dose is extremely small.

Nonetheless, even that very small amount of health-food-grade fish oil used in the mid-1980s was enough to cause significant gastric problems. No wonder the fish oil mania that swept our nation in the mid-1980s burned out so quickly. People were not seeing any perceptible health benefits because the amounts they were taking were too low to have any positive effect. Adding insult to injury, once the capsule dissolved in the stomach, many people were bothered by a fishy aftertaste on their breath for hours. If that wasn't enough, other contaminants (usually weird fatty acids made by algae) present in the fish oil would usually cause bloating and diarrhea.

Although the vitamin A was removed from the fish body oil capsules, there was still the lingering problem of PCBs and dioxins. To deal with this problem, some manufacturers employed a technology called molecular distillation, which removed some, but not all, of the PCBs and dioxins. Because molecular distillation also removed cholesterol, it was possible to market these fish oil products as cholesterol-free. (Actually they weren't, but the amount of cholesterol dropped below the limit required by the government to make that claim.)

The real breakthrough in fish oils occurred around 2000 with the advent of ultra-refined EPA/DHA concentrates. These required advanced chemical engineering that begins with the removal of most of the saturated fat by fractional distillation, as well as removing virtually all the PCBs (measured in parts per billion) and dioxins (measured in parts per trillion) by more sophisticated molecular distillation. With these innovations, a new type of fish oil was created, one that could deliver a concentrated amount of long-chain omega-3 fatty acids without unwanted by-products like chemical contaminants or harmful fatty acids. Basically, these new ultra-refined EPA/DHA concentrates could be considered weapons-grade fish oil: highly concentrated, highly purified, and ready for action.

Ultra-Refined EPA/DHA Concentrates

What are the standards for an ultra-refined EPA/DHA concentrate? There are four criteria that must be met. Unfortunately, most of these criteria do not have to be listed on a product label. This means you have to rely on the integrity of the brand, which is always risky in the health-food business.

The only thing that will usually appear on the label is the level of EPA and DHA. Even here, it is easy to be misled. Always look for at least 60 percent of the fatty acids consisting of EPA and DHA. Only concentrates above these levels of EPA and DHA have sufficient purity to usually meet the other three criteria. Although the other three criteria are never listed, here is what they should be:

PCBs	less than 30 parts per billion (ppb)
Dioxins	less than 1 part per trillion (ppt)
Total oxidation (Totox)	less than 20 meq/kg

These are very stringent conditions, and only a handful of the fish oil supplements sold can meet them. Let's see why each criterion is crucial for ensuring the potential benefits of an EPA/DHA concentrate in reducing inflammation.

First, natural fish oil contains only 5 to 20 percent of its fatty acids as a combination of EPA and DHA. The vast majority of the fatty acids in fish oil are primarily saturated fats, plus some monounsaturated fatty acids that are disruptive to your gastrointestinal tract. Your body wasn't meant to digest these fatty acids produced by algae. (Remember, fish don't make fish oil; they simply accumulate algae that makes EPA and DHA.) Removing them from fish oil can help prevent gastrointestinal distress without sacrificing any health benefits.

Second, crude fish oil should be considered the sewer of the sea. Anything that is fat-insoluble, such as PCBs, dioxins, and organic mercury compounds, will be found in the crude fish oil. To remove these chemicals requires extensive chemical processing because it usually takes 100 gallons of crude fish oil to make one gallon of an EPA/DHA concentrate. If these levels of PCBs are not stated to be less than 30 parts per billion (ppb), then the fish oil probably contains them. Here's a helpful hint: be very wary if a manufacturer states that the PCB levels are "below the limits of detection." This merely means that the detector they used is not very sensitive. Unfortunately, both your body and brain will detect them.

Third, the levels of total oxidation (Totox) of the fish oil, including peroxides, ketones, and aldehydes, are especially important since the aldehydes and ketones (both breakdown products of peroxides) can cause damage to your DNA. You can't smell peroxides, but it is the aldehydes and ketones that give fish its off-flavors. If a fish oil product smells "fishy," then it is more likely to cause damage to your DNA.

Judging the Quality of Fish Oil

Unless you have about $500,000 worth of testing equipment in your kitchen, you are not ever going to be able to determine how purified an EPA/DHA concentrate is. A manufacturer may state that fish oil is "pharmaceutical grade," but there is no standard definition for what this means. The laws that govern the supplement industry in the United States are extremely lax, allowing manufacturers to put whatever they want on a product label as long as it doesn't promise to cure or prevent a particular disease. Therefore, any fish oil that you purchase should be considered "buyer beware."

So what is a consumer to do? There are three options. The first is a simple test that I call the *toothpick test* to give you some indication of the approximate purity of the fish oil. Here it is: Pour a few teaspoonfuls of liquid fish oil into a shot glass and place it in your freezer for five hours. (If you have capsules, cut a few capsules in half and squeeze the liquid out.) Come back five hours later. If you can still pass a toothpick easily through the oil, then it might be okay. If the oil is frozen solid, then it's probably the sewer of the sea.

The second simple test is the smell and taste of the liquid fish oil itself. Humans have developed a sensitive system of taste and smell to indicate danger in eating a particular food item. Fish oil is no different.

If the taste of the fish oil is fishy, this is a strong indicator that significant "hidden oxidation" is already present. This fishy taste comes from oxidative breakdown products of the EPA and DHA known as aldehydes. These aldehydes can covalently bind to DNA, eventually causing breakage of the DNA.

Unfortunately, these two simple tests alone still won't tell you whether the product contains an unacceptable level of PCBs or dioxins, but it's a start.

The third option is to go to a free Web site run by an independent third party to see if the fish oil you are taking meets the standards I have outlined. The best Web site, in my opinion, is www.ifosprogram.com, which is run by the University of Guelph in Canada. IFOS (short for International Fish Oil Standards) uses the most sophisticated testing in the world to look for contaminants. Every fish oil lot that is tested is given a rating based on how well it does on the testing. As a consequence, many manufacturers never submit their oils for testing as all the results are posted on the Internet. Others might submit only one lot, letting you think that all lots they have produced are the same. (This is like thinking that every year of a wine vintage will always have the same taste.)

So what if the fish oil lot you are taking isn't listed on the site? The absence of any test results should make you highly suspect of its quality.

How Much Should You Spend?

To get the benefits of omega-3 fatty acids, you have to take a therapeutic dosage. Unfortunately, that is a lot higher than anyone ever anticipated. So you really have to consider the cost of EPA and DHA in the fish oil product. And here, potency is important. For lower-potency fish oils, the cost of the soft gelatin capsule is often much greater than the cost of the fish oil itself. So when you calculate the actual cost per gram of EPA and DHA that you are getting, it is really pretty expensive. Although purified EPA/DHA concentrates appear to cost more, the actual cost of the active ingredients (EPA and DHA) is often less. You should expect to pay about $0.60 per gram of EPA and DHA. So let's go back to my dosage chart described in chapter 9 and now add in the cost.

Condition	EPA and DHA required	Daily Cost
Maintain wellness	2.5 g/day	$1.50
Obesity, type 2 diabetes, heart disease, or before starting a diet	5 g/day	$3
Chronic pain	7.5 g/day	$4.50
Existing neurological conditions	10 g/day	$6

Here lies the unvarnished truth about nutritional supplements: to have them work, you need to take enough. Typically in the health-food industry, everything is done backward. They figure the most a customer will pay is about $5 to $15 per month. Then they put enough of a particular supplement in a bottle to meet that price point. No matter if the supplement actually works (and fish oil is one of the few supplements that meets that critera), if you don't take enough, you will not see the benefits.

Short-Chain Versus Long-Chain Omega-3 Fatty Acids

Not all omega-3 fatty acids are created equal. Only the long-chain omega-3 fatty acids, such as EPA, have the maximum impact on balancing your eicosanoid levels. Furthermore, DHA is a powerful activator of transcription factors and necessary for optimal brain function. You can only get these long-chain omega-3 fatty acids from fish oil. Short-chain omega-3 fatty acids such as alpha linolenic acid (ALA), found in flaxseed oil and other seed oils, have the potential to be made into their longer-chain relatives, such as EPA and DHA. The trouble is that the biosynthetic process is incredibly inefficient, and so you can't really get much long-chain fatty acids from short-chain ones. In fact, you would need to consume nearly 20 grams of ALA to make 1 gram of EPA and 0.1 gram of DHA. This is not a very good return on your dietary investment.

High-Dose EPA/DHA Concentrates: How Much Is Too Much?

Ultra-refined EPA/DHA concentrates only contain a few calories. Consuming a maintenance dose (2.5 grams of omega-3 fatty acids per day) will provide about an extra 35 calories a day. Even using 10 grams of long-chain omega-3 fatty acids per day using EPA/DHA concentrates would add less than 200 calories per day. The good news is that any increase in calories is more than balanced as it becomes easier to lose excess fat. The EPA in fish oil will inhibit the binding of endo-cannabinoids to their receptors (so you don't eat as much), and the DHA increases the expression of fat-burning enzymes by activating the PPAR-alpha transcription factor. One of the reasons that Manuel Uribe (the heaviest man in the world described in chapter 4) is losing so much weight is that he is taking about 20 grams of EPA and DHA per day. These levels not only decrease his hunger but also increase the metabolic use of stored fat.

The Safety of High-Dose Fish Oil

High-dose fish oil has been studied extensively for years in well-designed research trials and has been deemed to be extremely safe. Nonetheless, there remain many misconceptions about the use of high-dose fish oil. In an earlier book (*The OmegaRx Zone*), I described why these concerns are misplaced. As I have described in this book, the use of extremely high-dose fish oil (more than 15 grams of EPA and DHA per day) in children and adults is incredibly safe as long as the purity is excellent and you are using the AA/EPA ratio to determine the maximum dose to be used. At levels of 5 grams of EPA and DHA per day, there is no need for monitoring the blood as it is virtually impossible to get the AA/EPA ratio to be less than 1.5.

However, the use of high-dose fish oils does have one problem: reduction in the production of good eicosanoids because they inhibit dihomo-gamma-linolenic acid (DGLA) production. So taking high-dose fish oils *alone* in your war against silent inflammation is like taking two steps forward and one step back. You are still ahead in reducing pro-inflammation but have somewhat reduced your body's ultimate cellular rejuvenation capacity. In my own clinical trials as well as those done by others, you see a consistent outcome with high-dose fish oils: AA/EPA ratios are decreased, and the AA/DGLA ratios are usually increased.

Let me give you some examples from some of my own clinical trials as well as others:

Type of Study	EPA & DHA/day	Changes	Significance
Sleep-deprivation	2.5 g	AA/EPA -74 percent	$p < 0.001$
		AA/DGLA +93 percent	$p < 0.001$

Type of Study	EPA & DHA/day	Changes	Significance
Postmenopausal women	4 g	AA/EPA -86 percent	$p < 0.001$
		AA/DGLA +46 percent	$p < 0.001$
Severely obese adults	5 g	AA/EPA -69 percent	$p < 0.001$
		AA/DGLA +44 percent	$p < 0.004$

As you can see, every time with high-dose fish oil, the AA/EPA decreases (that's good), but the AA/DGLA increases (that's bad).

This means that if you are successfully reducing pro-inflammation, you are usually simultaneously reducing internal anti-inflammation. The only way to circumvent this problem is by using the super fish oils that I describe in chapter 9. Both fish oil and super fish oil will reduce silent inflammation, but only the use of super fish oil containing trace amounts of gamma-linolenic acid (GLA) will further slow the rate of aging.

Insulin Resistance: It All Starts in Your Adipose Tissue

I'VE FOUND THAT SURPRISINGLY FEW PHYSICIANS UNDERSTAND WHAT insulin resistance means, let alone what causes it. In the simplest terms, it means that the signal insulin is trying to communicate is not getting through to its target cell. It's like continually ringing a doorbell and not having anyone answer. As a result, blood glucose is not taken out of the bloodstream effectively. The pancreas compensates by producing more insulin (hyperinsulinemia) to drive blood glucose by brute force into its target cell. This increased insulin in the bloodstream, when combined with a large excess of omega-6 fatty acids, will lead to excess production of arachidonic acid (AA), which means increased silent inflammation.

What causes insulin resistance in any cell is inflammation, and the prime suspect is the inflammatory cytokine called TNF alpha. TNF alpha is one of the inflammatory cytobines produced when nuclear transcription factor NF-kappaB is activated. When it was first discovered in the mid-1990s that TNF alpha was associated with insulin resistance, there was a great deal of interest until researchers found TNF alpha levels to be about the same in the blood of both diabetics and non-diabetics. Furthermore, injected antibodies to TNF alpha appeared to have little impact on insulin resistance. So there was a mystery of how TNF alpha could rise in different places in the body without being elevated in the bloodstream.

I believe the answer to this paradox lies in the metastatic spread of toxic fat. To understand how, you have to go back to find the primary cause of insulin resistance in other cells, and that means going back to the adipose tissue.

It is often assumed that insulin resistance is primarily a problem of the muscle cells, but in reality, all cells have insulin receptors. That's why insulin resistance can be found in liver cells, brain cells, and even fat cells. And it is in the fat cells where I believe the story of insulin resistance really begins.

If you have healthy fat cells (good fat), excess AA can be stored in them, thus preventing adverse effects in other organs. It is only when the fat cells become progressively sicker (bad fat) and eventually die (due to AA toxicity) that AA begins leaking from your adipose tissue and starts to accelerate the development of the chronic diseases often associated with obesity—this is Toxic Fat Syndrome.

Although I discussed these concepts briefly earlier, it is worth the effort to understand the science behind not only why silent inflammation makes you fat but also how that increased fat can be a possible staging area for continued inflammatory assault on every organ in your body.

Adipose Tissue

Fat cells are highly specialized cells that collectively make up your adipose tissue, just like liver cells work together to form your liver. Your adipose tissue is the heaviest organ in the body (as if you couldn't guess). More importantly, your adipose tissue is just as vital to your survival as any organ because it controls the flow of high-octane fuel (fat) to make adenosine triphosphate (ATP) as well as prevents lipotoxicity.

The two most important mechanisms to ensure survival are the ability to withstand the stress of starvation and the ability to respond to infection by microbial invaders. In lesser-developed species such as the fruit fly, all these functions are tied together in what is known as the fat body. This fat body senses energy and nutrient availability, controls the metabolism of those nutrients, and finally coordinates immunological responses with its current metabolic status. Although they are separate organs, the adipose tissue, the immune system, and the liver still retain their ancient genetic roots. That is why today there remains a strong communication link between inflammatory and metabolic signaling pathways.

Inflammatory Responses Mediated by Macrophages

Among the key cells in the inflammatory response are macrophages, which are derived from circulating white blood cells. Although white blood cells themselves are benign, once they are transformed into macrophages, they become killing machines. The primary signals that activate these white cells to become macrophages are a group of pro-inflammatory eicosanoids (leukotrienes) derived from AA. The leukotrienes also act as vasodilating agents that let the newly transformed macrophages escape from the bloodstream and enter into the lymphatic system so that they can circulate to the target site. The same leukotrienes act as chemical flares that lead the macrophages to the battlefield.

Once at the site of inflammation, the macrophages unleash a formidable arsenal of weapons, including free radicals and inflammatory cytokines, in the hopes of destroying any of the invading organisms. They then finish the battle by consuming the debris so that no further inflammatory signals remain. But the macrophages are called off their attack only by the signaling of various anti-inflammatory eicosanoids. The primary anti-inflammatory signals come from anti-inflammatory eicosanoids, such as lipoxins, epi-lipoxins, and resolvins, as well as other DGLA-derived eicosanoids. It is only by shutting down the attack phase led by macrophages that cellular rejuvenation (healing) can begin to take place.

This tightly linked system of cellular destruction and cellular rejuvenation is the basis of wellness. The problem occurs when either the destruction phase is constantly turned on (as in silent inflammation), or the rejuvenation phase is not operating at peak efficiency. In either case, you age faster and develop chronic disease at an earlier age.

Circulating white blood cells are not the only source of macrophages. They can also be generated within the adipose tissue, one of the most concentrated sites of stem cells in the body. With the appropriate stimulus, they can be transformed into either new fat cells or new macrophages (remember the fat cells and immune cells share common genetic ancestors). More important, both fat cells and macrophages have another shared factor—the ability to bind and take up fatty acids.

Fat on Fire

It has always been amazing to me that with all the talk about obesity, how few times researchers have actually looked inside adipose tissue to see what's going on. When they finally did in 2003, they found that up to 50 percent of the fat mass in genetically bred obese animals consisted of macrophages. This means only one thing: the fat was "on fire," because when you find macrophages, you also find inflammation. Growing levels of silent inflammation in adipose tissue sets the stage for the adipose tissue starting the spread of inflammation throughout the body.

As I stated earlier, excess AA in any cell is highly toxic, and fat cells are not immune to this toxicity. If the levels of AA rise above a critical threshold level, that particular fat cell will become progressively sicker and then finally die, releasing all its stored fat. This represents the point that good fat becomes bad. This is a moment of severe local emergency because a lot of stored toxic AA is being released, and the only cells that can clean up this fatty mess are the macrophages. But unlike fat cells, macrophages have only a limited capacity to absorb excess fat, so there is a call for even more macrophages (both from the bloodstream and the transformation of adipose stem cells into more macrophages). Electron micrographs of these salvage operations can show a massive number of macrophages surrounding a single dying fat cell. With all those macrophages going to town on the dead fat cell, a lot of TNF alpha is being released, which generates insulin resistance in nearby healthy fat cells. Likewise, the macrophages release another inflammatory cytokine known as IL-6. But unlike TNF alpha, IL-6 can easily circulate in the bloodstream to be taken up by the liver, where it stimulates the production of C-reactive protein (CRP). This is why elevated CRP levels are associated with excess fat but only in those individuals who have insulin resistance.

One of the key roles for insulin in your fat cells is its ability to inhibit the release of stored fatty acids, which is why insulin can be considered a storage hormone. (Remember that insulin inhibits the hormone-sensitive lipase in the fat cells.) However, when insulin levels are low—as when you are sleeping—nothing inhibits the release of the fatty acids from the fat cells into the bloodstream. Good thing, because without that released fat going to your liver to be converted into glucose, your brain might not make it through the night.

These fatty acids being released are in the form of non-esterified fatty acids (NEFA). As long as the release of NEFA is being well regulated, there is a consistent flow of high-octane fuel to the liver for synthesis into glucose for the brain as well as ATP for the rest of the body. What controls that flow is the activity of the hormone-sensitive lipase. As insulin resistance develops in the fat cells, insulin can no longer regulate the outward flow of NEFA, and the liver can't metabolize all of this excess fat into lipoproteins. The excess NEFA is immediately taken up by other cells and converted into triglycerides in the form of lipid droplets for storage.

But if these lipid droplets in the cells are rich in AA, then what you have done is establish a very efficient transport system to bring a very inflammatory mediator (AA) from safe storage in the adipose tissue into the interior of different organs—where it can cause increased inflammation at new sites greatly distant from the fat cells. This is metastasis of toxic fat, just as a cancer cell metastasizes from its primary tumor to start new tumors in other parts of the body.

Lipotoxicity: Fat in All the Wrong Places

Only one cell in the body can tolerate large amounts of fat in the form of triglycerides: the fat cell. The brain is rich in fat, but mostly in the form of phospholipids and sphingolipids, the major constituents of all membranes. So when cells other than fat cells start accumulating excess fat as triglycerides, bad things begin to happen. One is the spread of insulin resistance.

Because NEFAs are toxic (they can act as detergents to solubilize cell membranes), once they get into a cell, if they are not immediately used as an energy source, they are transformed into triglycerides and stored as lipid droplets. If this occurs in any cell other than a fat cell, it is called *lipotoxicity*. One of the first places these lipid droplets accumulate is in the smooth muscle cells. If the NEFAs are rich in AA (very likely as it was excess AA that caused the fat cell death in the first place), then this newly transported AA in the lipid droplets in the smooth muscle cells is very likely to generate internal inflammation. This means increased activation of NF-kappaB and the production of more TNF alpha to cause disruption of insulin signaling in the smooth muscle cell. This gives rise to the classical insulin resistance associated with type 2 diabetes, even though it all originally started out as insulin resistance in the adipose tissue caused by AA-induced sickness and eventually death of otherwise healthy fat cells.

If insulin resistance develops in the muscle cells (the primary storage site for carbohydrates), this means that the pancreas is forced to continually pump out more insulin to try to bring down excess blood glucose levels (glucose is toxic at high levels). This excess insulin in the blood is called *hyperinsulinemia*. As long as the pancreas can continue to secrete increasing levels of insulin to reduce blood glucose levels, type 2 diabetes will not develop. However, hyperinsulinemia will cause metabolic syndrome, a cluster of conditions including low HDL, high triglycerides, and small low-density lipoprotein (LDL) particles—all ultimately caused by hyperinsulinemia in the blood. If untreated, metabolic syndrome usually develops into type 2 diabetes within eight to ten years.

Type 2 diabetes develops only when the beta cells (the cells that produce insulin) in the pancreas become compromised by lipotoxicity and start producing less insulin. When that occurs, blood glucose levels begin to rise rapidly, as the pancreas can no longer keep up with the growing demand for increased insulin production. This is the clinical definition of diabetes. Once you develop type 2 diabetes, you can figure your potential lifespan has decreased about ten to fifteen years.

The smooth muscle cells and pancreas are not the only cells that begin to accumulate lipid droplets. Other organs susceptible to lipotoxicity are the liver (giving rise to fatty liver and eventually nonalcoholic steatohepatitis or NASH) and the heart (giving rise to foam cells and eventually the growth of atherosclerotic plaques). This is why heart and liver disease are highly associated with type 2 diabetes, but not particularly well correlated with excess weight.

What You Have to Do to Live Longer and Better

To live longer and better, you have to reverse Toxic Fat Syndrome. To do so, you have to reduce silent inflammation throughout the body, but first and foremost in the adipose tissue, which is ground zero for launching the metastatic spread of toxic fat.

As long as silent inflammation is under control in the adipose tissue, there will not be widespread fat cell death, and thus no resulting surge of macrophages into the adipose tissue to try to clean up the damage. Without those macrophages, the levels of TNF alpha and IL-6 will fall dramatically. What you ideally need is something that can be directly targeted to the fat cells to reduce the inflammation and that has no toxic side effects. What will do this? Fish oils rich in eicosapentaenoic acid (EPA).

The best way to get into the fat cells is to be a fatty acid. The high levels of EPA will dilute the AA in the adipose tissue. Ironically, the more genetically prone you are to become obese (because of a fat trap), the faster the EPA can get transported into the inflamed adipose tissue to put out the fire. It has been demonstrated in animal studies that this is exactly what happens.

Regardless of your genetics, you are going to need large amounts of EPA and DHA (docosahexaenoic acid) to keep your fat from becoming inflamed if you are overweight or obese. The starting range is about 5 grams of EPA and DHA per day. Manuel Uribe (the world's heaviest man) has been consuming approximately 20 grams of EPA and DHA per day to bring his AA/EPA ratio in the blood down to less than 2. Once he did, his insulin resistance disappeared. At the same time, he was also reducing endocannabinoids in the brain, thus reducing his desire to eat.

It will only take you thirty days to reduce the silent inflammation in the fat cells to turn a malignant tumor into a benign tumor. It will take a much longer period of time to reduce the size of that benign tumor. Realistically, you should plan to lose about one pound of fat per week. This means reducing your calorie intake by about 500 calories per day. In fact, my clinical trials have demonstrated if you try to cut back the dietary calorie intake more than 500 calories below your resting metabolic rate (RMR), significant irritability sets in, which leads to a lack of dietary compliance.

A realistic minimum amount of calories is about 1,500 calories per day for the average male and about 1,200 calories per day for the average female. But if these calories are divided among low-glycemic carbohydrates (primarily vegetables and limited amounts of fruits), low-fat protein, and monounsaturated fat as described in the meals found in chapter 13, then you won't feel hungry or deprived. This balance of macronutrients allows you to shift from a glucose-burning metabolism to a fat-burning metabolism, which means more ATP generation for fewer incoming calories. That is exactly what the Zone Diet is designed for. It's really a way of eating without hunger or deprivation, designed to produce satiety as well as generating the maximum amount of ATP for the least number of dietary calories.

For increased satiety, take your fish oil right after the evening meal to further inhibit endocannabinoids in the brain from interacting with their receptors for the next four to six hours. This is a very effective way of preventing the nighttime munchies, a common weak point for dietary compliance.

Although it is the EPA in the fish oil that reduces inflammation in the fat cells and inhibits endocannaboids, the DHA is also important as it is an activator of PPAR-alpha, which increases the production of enzymes involved in beta-oxidation of fatty acids. At high enough concentrations, DHA helps you burn fat faster.

Finally, the eicosanoid PGE_1 (derived from DGLA), which is useful in reducing inflammation, also increases the release of stored fat. The end result is even faster fat loss, especially for those with a genetic fat trap.

The real goal is reducing the inflammation in the adipose tissue while simultaneously reducing the total fat load of the adipose tissue. A proven clinical approach is the use of the Zone Diet coupled with high-dose fish oil, and ideally high-dose super fish oil.

Nutrigenomics: How Diet Affects the Expression of Your Genes

SEVENTY YEARS AGO, ONE OF THE SUREST WAYS TO WIN A NOBEL Prize was to make some new discovery in nutrition. Today, one of the surest ways to win a Nobel Prize is for a new discovery in genomics, the study of gene expression. Surprisingly, both areas are related.

The more we understand the molecular biology of our genes, the more obvious the power of food ingredients to alter the expression of those genes. This is a powerful statement: it implies that our diet can be used to turn genes on and off. This is because the mechanisms for the expression of our genes have often been dependent on the presence of nutrients in the diet.

The research to unravel the human genome has shown how few

functional genes actually exist within our DNA. What makes humans more complex than other species is the ability to quickly turn these limited number of genes on and off with greater precision. In other words, we can change the expression of our genes more effectively than we can of other species. This is why the search for those gene targets that can be exploited to treat chronic disease is one of the areas of greatest interest in modern molecular biology. Many of these gene targets are proteins in the cell called gene transcription factors, which can be activated to turn on certain genes and turn off other genes, especially those involved in inflammation. The two most important from the dietary perspective are NF-kappaB (which turns the inflammatory response on) and PPAR-gamma (which can turn the inflammatory response off).

Understanding how our diet can affect these particular transcription factors goes back to understanding the most primitive component of our immune system, the innate immune system. It is considered primitive only because we share many of the same components of this part of our immune system with plants. It is only with the advent of the new analytical tools of molecular biology that we are able to realize how complex it really is.

This part of our immune system acts as an early warning system to detect microbial invasion by pattern recognition of certain fragments of microbes. If one of these parts is present and binds to the surface of certain receptors called *Toll-like* receptors, it sets in motion a complex series of events that leads to an escalation of silent inflammation to begin the attack phase of our inflammatory response. (The term *toll* comes from the German word meaning "weird." If these receptors are missing in fruit flies, they end up looking weird.)

One of the most highly studied of these Toll-like receptors is TLR-4, which binds a certain fragment of bacteria known as lipopolysaccharide or LPS. Once this bacteria fragment finds its Toll-like receptor (much like a hormone binding to its receptor), events are set in motion that activate NF-kappaB. This activated transcription factor then goes into the nucleus of the cells to signal for the increased synthesis of inflammatory proteins. As more of these inflammatory proteins are made, they begin to amplify the inflammatory response needed to attack potential bacterial invaders.

The major problem from a dietary perspective is that one of the components of LPS required for its initial binding to this Toll-like receptor is the saturated fatty acid attached to it. In fact, just adding saturated fats to the external environment of the cell can activate NF-kappaB. That's the bad news. This is why diets rich in saturated fats can be inflammatory. The good news is that long-chain omega-3 fatty acids, such as EPA (eicosapentaenoic acid) and DHA (docosahexaenoic acid), can inhibit this binding and prevent a dietary activation of the inflammatory response of the innate immune system by saturated fats that would result in increased silent inflammation.

Unfortunately for Americans, the levels of EPA and DHA have dramatically been reduced in our diet, and there has been a corresponding increase in saturated and trans fats (think doughnuts). As a result, more diet-induced silent inflammation is being generated because our primitive innate immune system isn't sophisticated enough to differentiate between a real microbial invasion and an imbalance in fat composition of our diets.

Another benefit is that EPA and DHA also inhibit the activation of NF-kappaB itself even if you are eating a lot of saturated fats. So besides affecting the balance of inflammatory eicosanoids, adequate intake of EPA and DHA can also significantly inhibit other molecular components of the inflammatory response, such as Toll-like receptors and NF-kappaB.

Polyphenols are another nutrient that can also reduce the activation of NF-kappaB and hence reduce silent inflammation. Remember, polyphenols are the chemicals that give fruits and vegetables their color. In high enough concentrations, these polyphenols can inhibit the activation of NF-kappaB. This is why diets rich in fruits and vegetables (like the Zone Diet) are more anti-inflammatory than diets whose primary source of carbohydrates (such as grains and starches) lack color.

Polyphenols are incredibly bitter-tasting compounds, and that's why they are found in low concentrations in fruits and vegetables. Think of an apple as an example. It's a well-known saying that, "An apple a day keeps the doctor away." So let's think about what is really in an apple. First, let's take out all of the water in an apple because it's unlikely that will keep the doctor away. Next, let's take out all the carbohydrates. It gets even smaller. Now let's remove all the fiber. What you have left is a very tiny amount of polyphenols that can inhibit inflammation, but they taste terrible. So you can see that you have to eat a lot of apples to get their anti-inflammatory benefits. (Note that chocolate also contains polyphenols, but they, too, are incredibly bitter. This is why companies add a lot of sugar and fat to hide their taste.)

Reservatrol is the polyphenol found in red grapes (not to mention red wine). It is likely that many of the health benefits of red wine come from this polyphenol. (Of course, the alcohol helps mask the bitter taste by dampening your taste receptors.) Recent experiments at Harvard indicate that if you give enough of this polyphenol (the equivalent of drinking about three hundred glasses of red wine per day) to obese rats, they live longer in spite of their obesity. The reason? Most likely the inhibition of NF-kappaB reduces silent inflammation and thus leads to a longer life.

Just to demonstrate that there is no one magical polyphenol

(remember there are probably more than 20,000), I combined a number of polyphenols from common fruits and vegetables and tested them against fat cells that had been stimulated by TNF to activate NF-kappaB. The results indicate that as you increase the concentration of these combined polyphenols, the amount of NF-kappaB that is activated in response to TNF can be dramatically reduced. This is essentially a high-tech validation of your grandmother's advice to eat your fruits and vegetables.

The other key component of fruits and vegetables that gives them anti-inflammatory actions is salicylates. These natural compounds also inhibit NF-kappaB. Salicylates are the compounds used by fruits and vegetables to defend themselves against microbial invaders, such as a virus. They help seal off areas of attack by causing cell death. The telltale sign that a fruit or vegetable has lots of salicylates inside is the number of dark spots on the surface. These dark spots (that is, bruises) seen on the surface of the fruit and vegetable are the result of past immunological struggles between the plant and microbial invaders. The more bruises a plant has indicate it has been gearing up its salicylate production. Since the advent of herbicides and pesticides some seventy years ago, plants don't have to work as hard in making salicylates. Thus we have grown accustomed to eating only fruits and vegetables that look like they came from central casting. Unfortunately, these fruits and vegetables usually contain 20 percent less salicylates than organically grown varieties that have to rely on themselves for protection against microbial invaders. The organic varieties don't look as nice in the supermarket, but they contain a lot more anti-inflammatory agents.

Remember that the most important anti-inflammatory drug we have today is aspirin. Like polyphenols, salicylates also taste terrible. This is why the biggest drug breakthrough in the nineteenth century was reducing the bitterness of salicylic acid by converting it to acetyl-salicylic (aspirin). Now it didn't taste so bad, and people could take an adequate dose to reduce inflammation. It is kind of like adding a lot of sugar and fat to the polyphenols in cocoa to make them taste better.

So why eat a lot of fruits and vegetables when it is just easier to take an aspirin? First, aspirin has a lot of side effects, such as bleeding, while fruits and vegetables do not. Second, aspirin doesn't contain any polyphenols. Third, if you are eating a lot of fruits and vegetables, it means you probably aren't eating a lot of grain and processed starches, thereby reducing insulin secretion. Finally, you are in dietary harmony with your genes because fruits and vegetables were the primary sources of carbohydrates for humans thousands of years ago. Our innate immune system was designed to have these food components as integral control points for the molecular modulation of inflammatory responses. When they are taken out of the diet and replaced by grains (that didn't exist ten thousand years ago), the result is increased silent inflammation.

However, this is not to say that aspirin doesn't have its benefits. Pioneering work by Charles N. Serhan at Harvard Medical School has shown that very low-dose aspirin can make a whole new series of incredibly powerful anti-inflammatory eicosanoids known as epi-lipoxins. But here is the problem: the more aspirin you take, the fewer of these epi-lipoxins are made. But if you combine high-dose fish oil with low-dose aspirin, you get another group of powerful anti-inflammatory eicosanoids known as resolvins. What's a low dose of aspirin? It's about one-half of a baby aspirin. So it is as if the wonder drug of the twentieth century (aspirin) is reaching out and joining forces with the wonder drug of the twenty-first century (high-dose fish oil) to make powerful compounds that help reduce inflammatory responses.

Just as NF-kappaB can turn on inflammation, another gene target can turn on anti-inflammation. These are the transcription factors known as perixosome proliferator activated receptors or PPAR for short. One subset of these receptors is PPAR-gamma. Once activated, it goes into the DNA to cause the synthesis of anti-inflammatory proteins, such as interleukin-10. Activation of PPAR-gamma in the fat cells also induces the synthesis of the hormone adiponectin that reduces insulin resistance. That's great news.

Unfortunately, the same gene products coming from the activation of PPAR-gamma also encourage production of new fat cells. But these new fat cells are healthy (good fat) and can encapsulate more arachidonic acid (AA), thus reducing the likelihood of Toxic Fat Syndrome. In essence, you get fatter but live longer (just like the fat rats who were consuming massive amounts of the polyphenol reservatol).

I hope you can see that the expression of many of our inflammatory genes to synthesize inflammatory proteins can be controlled by the food we eat. You can't change your genes, but you can definitely change their expression. The end result is decreased silent inflammation, and that means a longer and better life.

Zone Food Blocks

THE ZONE FOOD BLOCK METHOD IS THE MOST ACCURATE METHOD to determine the amount of carbohydrate you need at a meal because it takes into account the amount of fiber in the carbohydrate since fiber has no effect on insulin.

Simply use the hand-eye method to estimate the amount of protein you need at a meal, and then add a dash of heart-healthy monounsaturated fat. Now your only decision is how much carbohydrate to add to complete the meal. The typical female will have three Zone Carbohydrate Blocks at each meal; whereas the average male will have four Zone Carbohydrate Blocks at each meal.

The more low glycemic-load carbohydrates (nonstarchy vegetables) you consume, the larger the carbohydrate volume of each meal becomes. On the other hand, if you use high glycemic-load carbohydrates, such as grains, bread, and pasta, the emptier the plate is going to be. Unlike protein and fat, when people many times use only one item, you can add a variety of Zone Carbohydrate Blocks until they equal the amount you need for that meal. Try to get as much color out of your carbohydrates since that indicates they are rich in polyphenols.

Listed below are both low glycemic-load ("good") and high glycemic-load ("bad") Zone Carbohydrate Blocks. This illustrates the power of the Zone Diet: You never restrict anything from your plate, but treat high glycemic-load carbohydrates like condiments.

The guide will also come in handy when making substitutions in Zone meals. Don't want half an apple? Substitute 1 peach or half an orange or half a cup of grapes and so on. Likewise, don't like green beans? Instead of one and a half cups of green beans, have two cups of zucchini or one-quarter cup of kidney beans or two tomatoes. It's pretty easy to have an infinite variety of meals using the foods you like to eat.

Low Glycemic-Load Carbohydrates

Amount for one Zone Carbohydrate Block

Cooked vegetables

Artichoke	4 large
Artichoke hearts	1 cup
Asparagus	12 spears
Beans, black	1/4 cup
Beans, green or wax	1 1/2 cups
Bok choy	3 cups
Broccoli	4 cups

Brussel sprouts	1 1/2 cups
Cabbage	3 cups
Carrots, sliced	1 cup
Cauliflower	4 cups
Chickpeas	1/4 cup
Collard greens, chopped	2 cups
Eggplant	1 1/2 cups
Kale	2 cups
Kidney beans	1/4 cup
Leeks	1 cup
Lentils	1/4 cup
Mushrooms, boiled	2 cups
Okra, sliced	1 cup
Onions, chopped and boiled	1/2 cup
Sauerkraut	1 cup
Spaghetti squash	1 cup
Spinach, chopped	4 cups
Swiss chard, chopped	2 1/2 cups
Turnip, mashed	1 1/2 cups
Turnip greens, chopped	4 cups
Yellow squash, sliced	2 cups
Zucchini, sliced	2 cups

Raw vegetables

Alfalfa sprouts	10 cups
Bamboo shoots	4 cups
Bean sprouts	3 cups
Broccoli florets	4 cups

Cabbage, shredded	4 cups
Carrots, shredded	1 cup
Cauliflower florets	4 cups
Celery, sliced	2 cups
Cucumber	$1^1/_2$ medium
Cucumber, sliced	4 cups
Endive, chopped	10 cups
Escarole, chopped	10 cups
Green or red peppers	2
Green or red peppers, chopped	2 cups
Hummus	$^1/_4$ cup
Jalapeno peppers	2 cups
Lettuce, iceberg (6" diameter)	2 heads
Lettuce, romaine, chopped	10 cups
Mushrooms, chopped	4 cups
Onions, chopped	$1^1/_2$ cups
Radishes, sliced	4 cups
Salsa	$^1/_2$ cup
Snow peas	$1^1/_2$ cups
Spinach, chopped	10 cups
Tomato	2
Tomato, cherry	2 cups
Tomato, chopped	$1^1/_2$ cups
Water chestnuts	$^1/_2$ cup
Watercress	10 cups

Fruits

Apple (small)	$^1/_2$

Applesauce, unsweetened	$1/3$ cup
Apricots	3
Blackberries	$3/4$ cup
Boysenberries	$1/2$ cup
Cherries	8
Fruit cocktail, light	$1/3$ cup
Grapefruit	$1/2$
Grapes	$1/2$ cup
Kiwi	1
Lemon	1
Lime	1
Nectarine, medium	$1/2$
Orange	$1/2$
Orange, mandarin, canned in water	$1/3$
Peach	1
Peaches, canned in water	$1/2$
Pear	$1/2$
Plum	1
Raspberries	1 cup
Strawberries, diced fine	1 cup
Tangerine	1

Grains

Barley, dry	$1/8$ cup
Oatmeal, slow cooking	$1/3$ cup
Oatmeal, slow cooking, dry	1 ounce

Dairy (contains both a protein and carbohydrate block)

Milk (low-fat)	1 cup
Milk, soy	1 cup
Yogurt, plain	1/2 cup

High Glycemic-Load Carbohydrates

Amount for one Zone Carbohydrate Block

Cooked vegetables

Acorn squash	1/2 cup
Beans, baked	1/4 cup
Beans, refried	1/4 cup
Beets, sliced	1/2 cup
Butternut squash	1/2 cup
Corn	1/4 cup
French fries	5
Lima beans	1/4 cup
Parsnips	1/3 cup
Peas	1/2 cup
Pinto beans	1/4 cup
Potato, baked	1/4
Potato, boiled	1/3 cup
Potato, mashed	1/4 cup
Sweet potato, baked	1/3 cup
Sweet potato, mashed	1/4 cup

Fruits

Banana	$1/3$
Cantaloupe	$1/4$
Cantaloupe, cubed	$3/4$ cup
Cranberries	$3/4$ cup
Cranberry sauce	3 teaspoons
Fig	1
Guava	$1/2$
Honeydew melon, cubed	$2/3$ cup
Kumquat	3
Mango, sliced	$1/3$ cup
Papaya, cubed	$3/4$ cup
Pineapple, diced	$1/2$ cup
Prunes, dried	2
Raisins	1 tablespoon
Watermelon, cubed	$3/4$ cup

Fruit juices

Apple	$1/3$ cup
Apple cider	$1/3$ cup
Cranberry	$1/4$ cup
Fruit punch	$1/4$ cup
Grape	$1/4$ cup
Grapefruit	$1/3$ cup
Lemonade, unsweetened	$1/3$ cup
Lime	$1/3$ cup
Orange	$1/3$ cup

Pineapple	$^1/_4$ cup
Tomato	1 cup
V8 juice	$^3/_4$ cup

Grains, cereals, and breads

Bagel, small	$^1/_4$
Biscuit	$^1/_2$
Bread crumbs	$^1/_2$ ounce
Bread, whole grain or white	$^1/_2$ slice
Breadstick, hard	1
Breadstick, soft	$^1/_2$
Breakfast cereal, dry	$^1/_2$ ounce
Buckwheat, dry	$^1/_2$ ounce
Bulgur wheat, dry	$^1/_2$ ounce
Cornbread	$^1/_4$ square inch
Cornstarch	4 teaspoons
Couscous, dry	$^1/_2$ ounce
Cracker, graham	$1^1/_2$
Cracker, saltine	4
Cracker, Triscuit	3
Croissant, plain	$^1/_4$
English muffin	$^1/_4$
Granola	$^1/_2$ ounce
Grits, cooked	$^1/_3$ cup
Melba toast	$^1/_2$ ounce
Millet, dry	$^1/_2$ ounce
Muffin, blueberry mini	$^1/_2$
Noodles, egg, cooked	$^1/_4$ cup

Pancake, 4-inch	1
Pasta, cooked	$1/4$ cup
Pita bread	$1/2$ pocket
Pita bread, mini	1 pocket
Popcorn, popped	2 cups
Rice, brown, cooked	$1/5$ cup
Rice, white, cooked	$1/5$ cup
Rice cake	1
Roll, bulkie	$1/4$
Roll, hamburger	$1/2$
Roll, small dinner	$1/2$
Taco shell	1
Tortilla, 6-inch, corn	1
Tortilla, 8-inch, flour	$1/2$
Waffle	$1/2$

Alcohol

Beer, light	6 ounces
Beer, regular	4 ounces
Distilled spirits	1 ounce
Wine	4 ounces

Others

Barbeque sauce	2 tablespoons
Cake	$1/3$ slice
Candy bar	$1/4$
Catsup	2 tablespoons
Cocktail sauce	2 tablespoons

Cookie, small	1
Frozen tofu	1/6 cup
Honey	1/2 tablespoon
Ice cream, premium	1/6 cup
Ice cream, regular	1/4 cup
Jam or jelly	2 tablespoons
Molasses, light	1/2 teaspoon
Plum sauce	1 1/2 tablespoons
Potato chips	1/2 ounce
Pretzels	1/2 ounce
Sugar, brown	2 teaspoons
Sugar, confectionary	1 tablespoon
Sugar, cube	3
Sugar, granulated	2 teaspoons
Syrup, maple	2 teaspoons
Syrup, pancake	2 teaspoons
Teriyaki sauce	1 tablespoon
Tortilla chips	1/2 ounce

The Zone Diet Paradox

You can see that if you make all of your meals using low glycemic-load carbohydrates, you will be eating a large volume of food with relatively few calories. In fact, you would be consuming ten to fifteen servings of fruits and vegetables based on USDA portion sizes. That's three to five servings of fruits and vegetables per meal, and most Americans never consume more than two servings per day (usually french fries and catsup). Yet at the same time, you would also be consuming between 1,200 and 1,500 calories per day without hunger or deprivation.

On the other hand, consuming high glycemic-load carbohydrates will either leave a very empty plate (if you are consuming the right amount of Zone Carbohydrate Blocks) or produce excess insulin (if you are consuming the typical portion sizes of those high glycemic-load carbohydrates that most Americans do).

Zone Protein and Fat Blocks

Just for completeness, if you feel that some low-fat protein the size of your palm and a dash of fat is not rigorous enough for you, I have also included the corresponding Zone Food Block portions for both low-fat protein and good fat.

Zone Protein Blocks

Best Choices (low in saturated fat)

Beef (range-fed or game)	1 ounce
Chicken breast, deli-style	1 1/2 ounces
Chicken breast, skinless	1 ounce
Turkey, ground	1 1/2 ounces
Turkey breast, deli-style	1 1/2 ounces
Turkey breast, skinless	1 ounce

Fair Choices (moderate in saturated fat)

Beef, ground (less than 10% fat)	1 1/2 ounces
Beef, lean cut	1 ounce
Canadian bacon, lean	1 ounce
Chicken, dark meat, skinless	1 ounce
Corned beef, lean	1 ounce

Duck	1^1/$_2$ ounces
Ham, deli-style	1^1/$_2$ ounces
Ham, lean	1 ounce
Lamb, lean	1 ounce
Pork chop	1 ounce
Pork, lean	1 ounce
Turkey, dark meat, skinless	1 ounce
Turkey bacon	3 slices
Veal	1 ounce

Fish and Seafood

Bass, freshwater	1 ounce
Bass, sea	1^1/$_2$ ounces
Bluefish	1^1/$_2$ ounces
Calamari	1^1/$_2$ ounces
Catfish	1^1/$_2$ ounces
Clams	1^1/$_2$ ounces
Cod	1^1/$_2$ ounces
Crabmeat	1^1/$_2$ ounces
Haddock	1^1/$_2$ ounces
Halibut	1^1/$_2$ ounces
Lobster	1^1/$_2$ ounces
Mackerel	1^1/$_2$ ounces
Salmon	1^1/$_2$ ounces
Sardine	1 ounce
Scallops	1^1/$_2$ ounces
Shrimp	1^1/$_2$ ounces
Snapper	1^1/$_2$ ounces

Swordfish	1¹/2 ounces
Trout	1¹/2 ounces
Tuna (steak)	1 ounce
Tuna, canned in water	1 ounce

Eggs

Best Choices

| Egg substitute | ¹/4 cup |
| Egg whites (large) | 2 |

Protein-Rich Dairy

Best Choices

| Cheese, non-fat | 1 ounce |
| Cottage cheese, low fat | ¹/4 cup |

Fair Choices

Cheese, low fat	1 ounce
Mozzarella cheese, skim	1 ounce
Ricotta cheese, skim	2 ounces

Protein-Rich Vegetarian Choices (always check package labels)

Soy burgers	¹/2 patty
Soy hot dog	1 link
Soy sausage (links)	2 links
Soy sausage (patty)	1 patty
Soybean Canadian bacon	3 slices
Soybean frozen sausage	1 link

Soybean hamburger crumbles	1/2 cup
Soybean hotdog	1 link
Tofu, firm or extra firm	2 ounces

Zone Fat Blocks

Best Choices (rich in monounsaturated fat)

Almond, slivered	1 teaspoon
Almond butter	1/2 teaspoon
Almond Oil	1/3 teaspoon
Almonds, whole	3
Avocado	1 tablespoon
Cashews	2
Guacamole	1 tablespoon
Macadamia nuts	1
Olive oil	1/3 teaspoon
Olives	3
Peanut butter, natural	1 teaspoon
Peanut oil	1/3 teaspoon
Peanuts	6
Tahini	1/2 tablespoon

Fair Choices (low in saturated fat)

| Canola oil | 1/3 teaspoon |
| Walnuts, shelled and chopped | 1/2 teaspoon |

Glossary

Alpha-linolenic acid (ALA): The short-chain omega-3 fatty acid commonly found in the diet. Common sources include flaxseed and soy oils. The conversion of ALA into the longer-chain omega-3 fatty acids, such as EPA (eicosapentaenoic acid) and DHA (docosahexaenoic acid), is very inefficient in humans.

Anti-inflammatory medicine: Use of nutritional interventions to increase anti-inflammatory eicosanoids while simultaneously decreasing the production of pro-inflammatory eicosanoids.

Arachidonic acid (AA): Long-chain omega-6 fatty acid that is the immediate precursor of many eicosanoids that increase inflammation. Dietary sources include egg yolks, fatty red meat, and organ meats.

AA/DGLA ratio: Indicates balance of the precursors of pro-inflammatory to anti-inflammatory eicosanoids. The higher the AA/DGLA ratio, the fewer anti-inflammatory eicosanoids can be produced.

AA/EPA ratio: Determined from levels of long-chain omega-6 and omega-3 fatty acids. The AA/EPA ratio provides a precise measurement of the balance of eicosanoid precursors. The higher the AA/EPA ratio, the greater amount of silent inflammation.

COX (Cyclooxygenase): Enzyme required to convert essential fatty acids into prostaglandins and thromboxanes. There are two forms of this enzyme. The COX-1 enzyme is an integral part of many systems (like the cardiovascular system), whereas the COX-2 enzyme is inducible usually by activation of the NF-kappaB system during inflammation.

Dihomo-gamma-linolenic acid (DGLA): Essential fatty acid precursor of arachidonic acid. The eicosanoids derived from DGLA have powerful anti-inflammatory properties, unlike the pro-inflammatory properties of eicosanoids derived from AA. Adequate inhibition of the delta-5-desaturase will increase the levels of DGLA to AA in individual cells. There are no dietary sources that are rich in this essential fatty acid.

Docosahexaenoic acid (DHA): Long-chain omega-3 fatty acid that is critical for brain function; ultimately derived from EPA. DHA is found in high concentrations in fish oils.

Eicosanoids: Hormones derived from 20-carbon essential fatty acids AA, DGLA, and EPA, which control inflammation. The balance of eicosanoids that come from long-chain omega-3 and omega-6 essential fatty acids ultimately determine a person's state of wellness. The 1982

Nobel Prize in Medicine was awarded for understanding the role of eicosanoids in human disease.

Eicosapentaenoic acid (EPA): Long-chain omega-3 fatty acid that inhibits the formation of AA and also dilutes the presence of AA in the cell membrane. Fish oils are the richest source of EPA.

Endocannabinoids: Hormones derived from arachidonic acid that cause hunger once they bind to their receptors in the brain.

Essential fatty acids: Fatty acids that the body can't produce and, therefore, must be part of the diet. The two classes of essential fatty acids, omega-3 and omega-6, differ by the positions of the double bonds within the fatty acids. This positioning determines their three-dimensional structure in space, and hence the type of eicosanoids that can be made from them.

Gamma-linolenic acid (GLA): Immediate metabolic product of linoleic acid. This fatty acid is found in certain foods (such as oatmeal), edible oils (such as borage oil), and human breast milk. GLA is rapidly metabolized into DGLA and then potentially into AA, depending on the activity of the delta-5-desaturase enzyme.

Glucagon: Hormone stimulated by the protein content of a meal to cause the release of stored carbohydrates from the liver to help maintain blood glucose levels. It also decreases the activity of the delta-5-desaturase enzyme that produces arachidonic acid.

Insulin: Secreted by the beta cells of the pancreas to lower blood sugar levels. The glycemic load of a meal determines the extent of insulin secretion. It is essentially a storage hormone that drives macronutrients (carbohydrates, protein, and fat) into cells for immediate use or long-term storage. High levels of insulin activate the delta-5-desaturase enzyme, thus increasing AA levels.

Linoleic acid: Short-chain omega-6 fatty that can be converted into arachidonic acid (AA) via intermediates such as gamma-linolenic acid (GLA) and dihomo-gamma-linolenic acid (DGLA). Linoleic acid is the most common dietary form of all essential fatty acids. It is found in high concentrations in vegetables oils, such as soybean, corn, safflower, and sunflower oils.

Lipooxygenase (LOX): Enzymes required to make leukotrienes and lipoxins.

Lipotoxicity: Occurs when lipid droplets composed of triglycerides begin to deposit in organs other than the adipose tissue. Once this happens, organ function becomes compromised.

Peptide YY (PYY): Hormone released from the intestine by the protein content of a meal. It goes directly to the brain to cause satiety.

Resolvins: Class of anti-inflammatory eicosanoids derived from EPA and DHA that is created by the inhibition of the COX enzyme by low-dose aspirin.

Silent inflammation: Inflammation at the cellular level, below the perception of pain.

Toxic Fat Syndrome: Occurs when excess AA begins to appear in the bloodstream. It is best measured by the AA/EPA ratio.

Bibliography

Introduction

Mathers C, Ritu S, Salomon J, Murray CJ, and Lopez AD. "Healthy life expectancy in 191 countries." *Lancet* 357 (2001): 1685–1691.

Nolte E and McKee CM. "Measuring the health care of nations." *Health Affairs* 27 (2008): 58–71.

Sears B. *The Anti-Inflammation Zone*. New York: Regan Books, 2005.

———. *The OmegaRx Zone*. New York: Regan Books, 2002.

———. *The Zone*. New York: Regan Books, 1995.

World Health Organization, *World Health Report 2000*.

Chapter 1: The Real Epidemic Behind the Obesity Crisis

Sears B. *The Anti-Aging Zone*. New York: Regan Books, 1999.

———. *The Anti-Inflammation Zone*. New York: Regan Books, 2005.

———. *The OmegaRx Zone.* New York: Regan Books, 2002.

———. *The Zone.* New York: Regan Books, 1995.

Chapter 2: The Perfect Nutritional Storm

Cooper R, Cutler J, Desvigne-Nickens P, Fortmann SP, Friedman L, Havlik R, Hogelin G, Marler J, McGovern P, Morosco G, Mosca L, Pearson T, Stamler J, Stryer D, and Thom T. "Trends and disparities in coronary heart disease, stroke, and other cardiovascular diseases in the United States: findings of the national conference on cardiovascular disease prevention." *Circulation* 102 (2000): 3137–3147.

Hossain P, Kawar B, and Nahas ME. "Obesity and diabetes in the developing world." *New England Journal of Medicine* 356 (2007): 213–216.

Katic M, and Kahn CR. "The role of insulin and IGF-1 signaling in longevity." *Cellular and Molecular Life Sciences* 62 (2005): 320–343.

Nestle M. *Food Politics.* Berkeley: University of California Press, 2002.

———. *What to Eat.* New York: North Point Press, 2006.

Pollan M. *The Omnivore's Dilemma.* New York: Penguin Press, 2006.

Sears B. *The Anti-Aging Zone.* New York: Regan Books, 1999.

———. *The OmegaRx Zone.* New York: Regan Books, 2002.

———. *The Zone.* New York: Reagan Books, 1995.

Simopoulos A and Robinson J. *The Omega Plan.* New York: Harper Collins, 1998.

Tatar M, Bartke A, and Antebi A. "The endocrine regulation of aging by insulin-like signals." *Science* 299 (2003): 1346–1351.

Yam D, Elitaz B, Eliraz B, and Elliot M. "Diet and disease: the Israeli paradox: possible dangers of a high omega-6 polyunsaturated fatty acid diet." *Israel Journal of Medical Sciences* 32 (1996): 1134–1143.

Chapter 3: How Inflammation Helps Us—and Hurts Us

Babcok T, Helton WS, and Espat NJ. "Eicosapentaenoic acid: an anti-inflammatory omega-3 fat with potential clinical applications." *Nutrition* 16 (2000): 1116–1118.

Bazan NG and Flower RL. "Lipid signals in pain control." *Nature* 420 (2002): 135–138.

Bibliography

Bechoua S, Dubois M, Nemoz G, Chapy P, Vericel E, Lagarde M, and Prigent AF. "Very low dietary intake of n-3 fatty acids affects the immune function of healthy elderly people." *Lipids* 34 (1999): S143.

Bleumink GS, Feenstra J, Sturkenboom MCMJ, and Stricker BHC. "Nonsteroidal anti-inflammatory drugs and heart failure." *Drugs* 63 (2003): 525–534.

Brenner RR. "Nutrition and hormonal factors influencing desaturation of essential fatty acids." *Progress in Lipid Research* 20 (1982): 41–48.

Calder PC. "n-3 polyunsaturated fatty acids and cytokine production in health and disease." *Annals of Nutrition and Metabolism* 41 (1997): 203–234.

———. "n-3 polyunsaturated fatty acids, inflammation and immunity." *Nutrition Research* 21 (2001): 309–341.

———. "Dietary modification of inflammation with lipids." *Proceedings of the Nutrition Society* 61 (2002): 345–358.

el Boustani S, Causse JE, Descomps B, Monnier L, Mendy F, and Crastes de Paulet A. "Direct in vivo characterization of delta-5-desaturase activity in humans by deuterium labeling: effect of insulin." *Metabolism* 38 (1989): 315–321.

Endres S. "Messengers and mediators: interactions among lipids, eicosanoids, and cytokines." *American Journal of Clinical Nutrition* 57 (1993): 798S–800S.

———. "n-3 polyunsaturated fatty acids and human cytokine synthesis." *Lipids* 31 (1996): S239–242.

Endres S and von Schacky C. "n-3 polyunsaturated fatty acids and human cytokine synthesis." *Current Opinion in Lipidology* 7 (1996): 48–52.

Endres S, Ghorbani R, Kelley VE, Georgilis K, Lonnemann G, van der Meer JW, Cannon JG, Rogers TS, Klempner MS, and Weber PC. "The effect of dietary supplementation with n-3 polyunsaturated fatty acids on the synthesis of interleukin-1 and tumor necrosis factor by mononuclear cells." *New England Journal of Medicine* 320 (1989): 265–271.

Harris JI, Hibbeln JR, Mackey RH, and Muldoon MF. "Statin treatment alters serum n-3 and n-6 fatty acids in hypercholestemic patients." *Prostaglandins, Leukotrienes and Essential Fatty Acids* 71 (2004): 263–269.

Hill EG, Johnson SB, Lawson LD, Mahfouz MM, and Holman RT. "Perturbation of the metabolism of essential fatty acids by dietary partially hydrogenated vegetable oil." *Proceedings of the National Academy of Sciences (USA)* 79 (1982): 953–957.

Lawrence T, Willoughby DA, and Gilroy DW. "Anti-inflammatory lipid mediators and insights into the resolution of inflammation." *Nature Reviews Immunology* 2 (2002): 787–795.

Levy B, Clish CB, Schmidt B, Gronert K, and Serhan CN. "Lipid mediator class switching during acute inflammation: signals in resolution." *Nature Reviews Immunology* 2 (2001): 612–619.

Lo CJ, Chiu KC, Fu M, Lo R, and Helton S. "Fish oil decreases macrophage tumor necrosis factor gene transcription by altering the NF-kappaB activity." *Journal of Surgical Research* 82 (1999): 216–221.

Mukherjee D, Nissen SE, and Topol EJ. "Risk of cardiovascular events associated with selective COX-2 inhibitors." *JAMA* 286 (2001): 954–959.

Oates JA. "The 1982 Nobel prize in physiology or medicine." *Science* 218 (1982): 765–768.

Sears B. *The Anti-Inflammation Zone.* New York: Regan Books, 2005.

———. *The OmegaRx Zone.* New York: Regan Books, 2002.

———. *The Zone.* New York: Regan Books, 1995.

Serhan CN, Hong S, Gronert K, Colgan SP, Devchand PR, Mirick G, and Moussignac RL. "Resolvins: a family of bioactive products of omega-3 fatty acid transformation circuits initiated by aspirin treatment that counter proinflammation signals." *Journal of Experimental Medicine* 196 (2002): 1025–1037.

Taubes, G. *Good Calories, Bad Calories.* New York: Alfred Knopf, 2007.

Trowbridge HO and Emling RC. *Inflammation. A Review of the Process—5th Edition.* Chicago: Quintessence Books, 1997.

Tsiotou AG, Sakorafas GH, Anagnostopoulos G, and Bramis J. "Septic shock; current pathogenetic concepts from a clinical perspective." *Medical Science Monitor* 11 (2005): 76–85.

Van Dyke TE and Serhan CN. "Resolution of inflammation." *Journal of Dental Research* 82 (2003): 82–90.

Wolfe M, Lichtenstein DR, and Singh G. "Gastrointestinal toxicity of nonsteroidal anti-inflammatory drugs." *New England Journal of Medicine* 340 (1999):1888–1899.

Bibliography

Zurier RB. "Eicosanoids and inflammation." *Prostaglandins in Clinical Practice*, edited by Watkins WD, Peterson MB, and Fletcher JR. New York: Raven Press, 1989.

Chapter 4: Why Getting Fat May Not Be Your Fault

Batterham RL, Cohen MA, Ellis SM, Le Roux CW, Withers DJ, Frost GS, Ghatei MA, and Bloom SR. "Inhibition of food intake in obese subjects by peptide YY." *New England Journal of Medicine* 349 (2003): 941–948.

Batterham RL, Heffron H, Kapoor S, Chivers JE, Chandarana K, Herzog H, Le Roux CW, Thomas EL, Bell JD, and Withers DJ. "Critical role for peptide YY in protein-mediated satiation and body-weight regulation." *Cell Metabolism* 4 (2006): 223–233.

Bluher M, Kahn BB, and Kahn CR. "Extended longevity in mice lacking the insulin receptor in adipose tissue." *Science* 299 (2003): 572–574.

Boord JB, Maeda K, Makowski L, Babaev VR, Fazio S, Linton MF, and Hotamisligil GS. "Combined adipocyte-macrophage fatty acid-binding protein deficiency improves metabolism, atherosclerosis, and survival in apolipoprotein E-deficient mice." *Circulation* 110 (2004): 1492–1498.

Botion LM and Green A. "Long-term regulation of lipolysis and hormone-sensitive lipase by insulin and glucose." *Diabetes* 48 (1999): 1691–1697.

Caballero B, Clay T, Davis SM, Ethelbah B, Rock BH, Lohman T, Norman J, Story M, Stone EJ, Stephenson L, and Stevens J. "Pathways: a school-based, randomized controlled trial for the prevention of obesity in American Indian schoolchildren." *American Journal of Clinical Nutrition* 78 (2003): 1030–1038.

Campos P. *The Obesity Myth*. New York: Gotham Books, 2004.

Cshe K, Winkler G, Melczer Z, and Baranyi E. "The role of tumor necrosis factor resistance in obesity and insulin resistance." *Diabetologia* 43 (2000): 525.

Despres JP. "The endocannabinoid system: a new target for the regulation of energy balance and metabolism." *Critical Pathways in Cardiology* 6 (2007): 46–50.

Ellacott KL, Halatchev IG, and Cone RD. "Interactions between gut peptides and the central melanocortin system in the regulation of energy homeostasis." *Peptides* 27 (2006): 340–349.

Engeili S, Bohnke J, Feldpausch M, Gorzelniak K, Janke J, Batkai S, Pacher P, Harvey-White J, Luft FC, Sharma AM, and Jordon J. "Activation of the peripheral endocannabinoid system in human obesity." *Diabetes* 54 (2005): 2838–2843.

Erbay E, Cao H, and Hotamisligil GS. "Adipocyte/macrophage fatty acid binding proteins in metabolic syndrome." *Current Atherosclerosis Reports* 9 (2007): 222–229.

Festa A, D'Agostino R, Howard G, Mykkanen L, Tracy RP, and Haffner SM. "Chronic subclinical inflammation as part of the insulin resistance syndrome." *Circulation* 102 (2000): 42–47.

Fruhbeck G, Gomez-Ambrosi J, Muruzabal FJ, and Burrell MA. "The adipocyte: a model for integration of endocrine and metabolic signaling in energy metabolism regulation." *American Journal of Physiology: Endocrinology and Metabolism* 280 (2001): E827–E847.

Haemmerle G, Zimmermann R, and Zechner R. "Letting lipids go: hormone-sensitive lipase." *Current Opinion in Lipidology* 14 (2003): 289–297.

Huda MS, Wilding JP, and Pinkney JH. "Gut peptides and the regulation of appetite." *Obesity Reviews* 7 (2006): 163–182.

Kekwick A and Pawar GLS. "Calorie intake in relation to body weight changes in the obese." *Lancet* ii (1956): 155–161.

————. "Metabolic study in human obesity with isocaloric diets high in fat, protein and carbohydrate." *Metabolism* 6 (1957): 447–460.

Kokot F and Ficek R. "Effects of neuropeptide Y on appetite." *Mineral and Electrolyte Metabolism* 25 (1999): 303–305.

Kolata G. *Rethinking Thin*. New York: Farrar, Straus, and Giroux, 2006.

Lee YH and Pratley RE. "The evolving role of inflammation in obesity and the metabolic syndrome." *Current Diabetes Reports* 5 (2005): 70–75.

Le Roux CW, Batterham RL, Aylwin SJ, Patterson M, Borg CM, Wynne KJ, Kent A, Vincent RP, Gardiner J, Ghatei MA, and Bloom SR. "Attenuated peptide YY release in obese subjects is associated with reduced satiety." *Endocrinology 2006* 147 (2006): 3–8.

Moran O and Phillip M. "Leptin: obesity, diabetes and other peripheral effects—a review." *Pediatric Diabetes* 4 (2003): 101–109.

Murphy KG and Bloom SR. "Gut hormones and the regulation of energy homeostasis." *Nature* 444 (2006): 854–859.

Musami SK, Erickson S, and Allison DB. "Obesity—still highly heritable after all these years." *American Journal of Clinical Nutrition* 87 (2008): 275–276.

Bibliography

Nader PR, Stone EJ, Lytle LA, Perry CL, Osganian SK, Kelder S, Webber LS, Elder JP, Montgomery D, Feldman HA, Wu M, Johnson C, Parcel GS, and Luepker RV. "Three-year maintenance of improved diet and physical activity: the CATCH cohort. Child and Adolescent Trial for Cardiovascular Health." *Archives of Pediatrics and Adolescent Medicine* 153 (1999): 695–704.

Naslund E and Hellstrom PM. "Appetite signaling: from gut peptides and enteric nerves to brain." *Physiology and Behavior* 92 (2007): 256–262.

Natali A and Ferrannini E. "Hypertension, insulin resistance, and the metabolic syndrome." *Endocrinology Metabolism Clinics of North America* 33 (2004): 417–429.

Oliver JE. *Fat Politics*. New York: Oxford University Press, 2006.

Osei-Hyiaman D, Harvey-White J, Batkai S, and Kunos G. "The role of the endo-cannabinoid system in the control of energy homeostasis." *International Journal of Obesity* 30 (2006): S33–38.

Qi K, Hall M, and Deckelbaum RJ. "Long-chain polyunsaturated fatty acid accretion in brain." *Current Opinion in Clinical Nutrition and Metabolic Care* 5 (2002): 133–138.

Pompeia C, Lima T, and Curi R. "Arachidonic acid cytotoxicity: Can arachidonic acid be a physiological mediator of cell death?" *Cell Biochemistry and Function* 21 (2003): 97–104.

Robertson RP and Harmon JS. "Diabetes, glucose toxicity, and oxidative stress: A case of double jeopardy for the pancreatic islet beta cell." *Free Radical Biology and Medicine* 41 (2006): 177–184.

Schwartz MW and Morton GJ. "Keeping hunger at bay." *Nature* 418 (2002): 595–597.

Schwartz MW and Porte D. "Diabetes, obesity, and the brain." *Science* 307 (2005): 375–379.

Sears B. *The Zone*. New York: Regan Books, 1995.

Silha JV, Krsek M, Skrha JV, Sucharda P, Nyomba BL, and Murphy LJ. "Plasma resistin, adiponectin and leptin levels in lean and obese subjects: correlations with insulin resistance." *European Journal of Endocrinology* 149 (2003): 331–335.

Small CJ and Bloom SR. "Gut hormones and the control of appetite." *Trends in Endocrinology and Metabolism* 15 (2004): 259–263.

Taubes G. *Good Calories, Bad Calories*. New York: Alfred Knopf, 2007.

Ukkola O. "Peripheral regulation of food intake: new insights." *Journal of Endocrinological Investigation* 27 (2004): 96–98.

van den Hoek AM, Teusink B, Voshol PJ, Havekes LM, Romijn JA, and Pijl H. "Leptin deficiency per se dictates body composition and insulin action in ob/ob mice." *Journal of Neuroendocrinology* 20 (2008): 120–127.

Wardle J, Carnell S, Haworth CMA, and Plomin R. "Evidence for a strong genetic influence on childhood adiposity despite the force of the obeseogeneic environment." *American Journal of Clinical Nutrition* 87 (2008): 398–404.

Yeaman SJ. "Hormone-sensitive lipase—new roles for an old enzyme." *Biochemical Journal* 379 (2004): 11–22.

Yudkin JS. "Inflammation, obesity, and the metabolic syndrome." *Hormone and Metabolic Research* 39 (2007): 707–709.

Chapter 5: Good Fat May Be Protective

Baylin A and Campos H. "Arachidonic acid in adipose tissue is associated with nonfatal acute myocardial infarction in the central valley of Costa Rica." *Journal of Nutrition* 134 (2004): 3095–3099.

Belanger MC, Dewailly E, Berthiaume L, Noel M, Bergeron J, Mirault ME, and Julien P. "Dietary contaminants and oxidative stress in Inuit of Nunavik." *Metabolism* 55 (2006): 989–995.

Bluher M, Engeli S, Kloting N, Berndt J, Fasshauer M, Batkai S, Pacher P, Schon MR, Jordan J, and Stumvoll M. "Dysregulation of the peripheral and adipose tissue endocannabinoid system in human abdominal obesity." *Diabetes* 55 (2006): 3053–3060.

Booth GL, Kapral MK, Fung K, and Tu JV. "Relation between age and cardiovascular disease in men and women with diabetes compared with non-diabetic people: a population-based retrospective cohort study." *Lancet* 368 (2006): 29–36.

Brochu M, Tchernof A, Dionne IJ, Sites CK, Eltabbakh GH, Sims EA, and Poehlman ET. "What are the physical characteristics associated with a normal metabolic profile despite a high level of obesity in postmenopausal women?" *Journal of Clinical Endocrinology and Metabolism* 86 (2001): 1020–1025.

Campos P. *The Obesity Myth*. New York: Gotham Books, 2004.

Flegal KM, Graubard BI, Williamson DF, and Gail MH. "Excess deaths associated with underweight, overweight, and obesity." *JAMA* 293 (2005): 1861–1867.

Bibliography

Flegal KM, Graubard BI, Williamson DF, and Gail MH. "Cause-specific excess deaths associated with underweight, overweight, and obesity." *JAMA* 298 (2007): 2028–2037.

Fonarow GC, Srikanthan P, Costanzo MR, Cintron GB, and Lopatin M. "An obesity paradox in acute heart failure: analysis of body mass index and in hospital mortality for 108,927 patients in the Acute Decompensated Heart Failure National Registry." *American Heart Journal* 153 (2007): 74–81.

Fontana L, Meyer TE, Klein S, and Holloszy JO. "Long-term calorie restriction is highly effective in reducing the risk for atherosclerosis in humans." *Proceedings of the National Academy of Sciences (USA)* 101 (2004): 6659–6663.

Iacobellis G, Ribaudo MC, Zappaterreno A, Iannucci CV, and Leonetti F. "Prevalence of uncomplicated obesity in an Italian obese population." *Obesity* 13 (2005): 1116–1122.

Karelis AD, Brochu M, and Rabasa-Lhoret R. "Can we identify metabolically healthy but obese individuals (MHO)?" *Diabetes and Metabolism* 30 (2004): 569–572.

Karelis AD, Faraj M, Bastard JP, St-Pierre DH, Brochu M, Prud'homme D, and Rabasa-Lhoret R. "The metabolically healthy but obese individual presents a favorable inflammation profile." *Journal of Clinical Endocrinology and Metabolism* 90 (2005): 4145–4150.

Kark JD, Kaufmann NA, Binka F, Goldberger N, and Berry EM. "Adipose tissue n-6 fatty acids and acute myocardial infarction in a population consuming a diet high in polyunsaturated fatty acids." *American Journal of Clinical Nutrition* 77 (2003): 796–802.

Knutson KL, Spiegel K, Penev P, and Van Cauter E. "The metabolic consequences of sleep deprivation." *Sleep Medicine Reviews* 11 (2007): 163–178.

Kolata G. *Rethinking Thin.* New York: Farrar, Straus, and Giroux, 2006.

Lecka-Czernik B, Moerman EJ, Grant DF, Lehmann JM, Manolagas SC, and Jilka RL. "Divergent effects of selective peroxisome proliferator-activated receptor-gamma 2 ligands on adipocyte versus osteoblast differentiation." *Endocrinology* 143 (2002): 2376–2384.

Lee WJ, Huang MT, Wang W, Lin CM, Chen TC, and Lai IR. "Effects of obesity surgery on the metabolic syndrome." *Archives of Surgery* 139 (2004): 1088–1092.

Massiera F, Saint-Marc P, Seydoux J, Murata T, Kobayashi T, Narumiya S, Guesnet P,

Amri EZ, Negrel R, and Ailhaud G. "Arachidonic acid and prostacyclin signaling promote adipose tissue development: a human health concern?" *Journal of Lipid Research* 44 (2003): 271–279.

Mazid MA, Chowdhury AA, Nagao K, Nishimura K, Jisaka M, Nagaya T, and Yokota K. "Endogenous 15-deoxy-delta(12, 14)-prostaglandin J(2) synthesized by adipocytes during maturation phase contributes to upregulation of fat storage." *FEBS Letters* 580 (2006): 6885–6890.

Oliver JE. *Fat Politics*. New York: Oxford University Press, 2006.

Petreas M, Smith D, Hurley S, Jeffrey SS, Gilliss D, and Reynolds P. "Distribution of persistent, lipid-soluble chemicals in breast and abdominal adipose tissues: lessons learned from a breast cancer study." *Cancer Epidemiology Biomarkers and Prevention* 13 (2004): 416–424.

Phelan S, Wyatt HR, Hill JO, and Wing RR. "Are the eating and exercise habits of successful weight losers changing?" *Obesity* 14 (2006): 710–716.

Robertson RP and Harmon JS. "Diabetes, glucose toxicity, and oxidative stress: A case of double jeopardy for the pancreatic islet beta cell." *Free Radical Biology and Medicine* 41 (2006): 177–184.

Romero-Corral A, Montori VM, Somers VK, Korinek J, Thomas RJ, Allison TG, Mookadam F, and Lopez-Jimenez F. "Association of bodyweight with total mortality and with cardiovascular events in coronary artery disease: a systematic review of cohort studies." *Lancet* 368 (2006): 666–678.

Savva SC, Chadjigeorgiou C, Hatzis C, Kyriakakis M, Tsimbinos G, Tornaritis M, and Kafatos A. "Association of adipose tissue arachidonic acid content with BMI and overweight status in children from Cyprus and Crete." *British Journal of Nutrition* 91 (2004): 643–649.

Sears B. *The Anti-Aging Zone*. New York: Regan Books, 1999.

Seyberth HW, Oelz O, Kennedy T, Sweetman BJ, Danon A, Frolich JC, Heimberg M, and Oates JA. "Increased arachidonate in lipids after administration to man: effects on prostaglandin biosynthesis." *Clinical Pharmacology and Therapeutics* 18 (1975): 521–529.

Silver MJ, Hoch W, Kocsis JJ, Ingerman CM, and Smith JB. "Arachidonic acid causes sudden death in rabbits." *Science* 183 (1974): 1085–1087.

Spiegel K, Leproult R, and Van Cauter E. "Impact of sleep debt on metabolic and endocrine function." *Lancet* 354 (1999): 1435–1439.

Bibliography

Unger RH. "Lipotoxic diseases." *Annual Review of Medicine* 53 (2002): 319–336.

———. "Longevity, lipotoxicity and leptin: the adipocyte defense against feasting and famine." *Biochimie* 87 (2005): 57–64.

Williams ES, Baylin A, and Campos H. "Adipose tissue arachidonic acid and the metabolic syndrome in Costa Rican adults." *Clinical Nutrition* 26 (2007): 474–482.

Wing RR and Hill JO. "Successful weight loss maintenance." *Annual Review of Nutrition* 21 (2001): 323–341.

Chapter 6: Malignant Toxic Fat

Aldamiz-Echevarria L, Prieto JA, Andrade F, Elorz J, Sanjurjo P, and Rodriguez Soriano J. "Arachidonic acid content in adipose tissue is associated with insulin resistance in healthy children." *Journal of Pediatric Gastroenterology and Nutrition* 44 (2007): 77–83.

Baylin A. and Campos H. "Arachidonic acid in adipose tissue is associated with nonfatal acute myocardial infarction in the central valley of Costa Rica." *Journal of Nutrition* 134 (2004): 3095–3099.

Chevrier J, Dewailly E, Ayotte P, Mauriege P, Despres JP, and Tremblay A. "Body weight loss increases plasma and adipose tissue concentrations of potentially toxic pollutants in obese individuals." *International Journal of Obesity and Related Metabolic Disorders* 24 (2000): 1272–1278.

Cinti S, Mitchell G, Barbatelli G, Murano I, Ceresi E, Faloia E, Wang S, Fortier M, Greenberg AS, and Obin MS. "Adipocyte death defines macrophage localization and function in adipose tissue of obese mice and humans." *Journal of Lipid Research* 46 (2005): 2347–2355.

Fox CS, Pencina MJ, Meigs JB, Vasan RS, Levitzky YS, and D'Agostino RB. "Trends in the incidence of type 2 diabetes mellitus from the 1970s to the 1990s: The Framingham Heart Study." *Circulation* 113 (2006): 2914–2918.

Huber J, Loffler M, Bilban M, Reimers M, Kadl A, Todoric J, Zeyda M, Geyeregger R, Schreiner M, Weichhart T, Leitinger N, Waldhausl W, and Stulnig TM. "Prevention of high-fat diet-induced adipose tissue remodeling in obese diabetic mice by n-3 polyunsaturated fatty acids." *International Journal of Obesity* 31 (2007): 1004–1013.

Hue O, Marcotte J, Berrigan F, Simoneau M, Dore J, Marceau P, Marceau S, Tremblay A, and Teasdale N. "Increased plasma levels of toxic pollutants accompanying weight loss induced by hypocaloric diet or by bariatric surgery." *Obesity Surgery* 16 (2006): 1145–1154.

Lelliott C and Vidal-Puig AJ. "Lipotoxcity, an imbalance between lipogenesis de novo and fatty acid oxidation." *International Journal of Obesity and Related Metabolic Disorders* 28 Suppl 4 (2004): S22–28.

Mazid MA, Chowdhury AA, Nagao K, Nishimura K, Jisaka M, Nagaya T, and Yokota K. "Endogenous 15-deoxy-delta(12, 14)-prostaglandin J(2) synthesized by adipocytes during maturation phase contributes to upregulation of fat storage." *FEBS Letters* 580 (2006): 6885–6890.

McLaughlin T, Sherman A, Tsao P, Gonzalez O, Yee G, Lamendola C, Reaven GM, and Cushman SW. "Enhanced proportion of small adipose cells in insulin-resistant vs insulin-sensitive obese individuals implicates impaired adipogenesis." *Diabetologia* 50 (2007): 1707–1715.

Pelletier C, Doucet E, Imbeault P, and Tremblay A. "Associations between weight loss-induced changes in plasma organochlorine concentrations, serum T(3) concentration, and resting metabolic rate." *Toxicology Sciences* 67 (2002): 46–51.

Petersen KF and Shulman GI. "New insights into the pathogenesis of insulin resistance in humans using magnetic resonance spectroscopy." *Obesity* 14 (2006): 34S–40S.

Phinney SD, Davis PG, Johnson SB, and Holman RT. "Obesity and weight loss alter serum polyunsaturated lipids in humans." *American Journal of Clinical Nutrition* 53 (1991): 831–838.

Pompcia C, Freitas JJ, Kim JS, Zyngier SB, and Curi R. "Arachidonic acid cytotoxicity in leukocytes: implications of oxidative stress and eicosanoid synthesis." *Biology of the Cell* 94 (2002): 251–265.

Pompeia C, Lima T, and Curi R. "Arachidonic acid cytotoxicity: can arachidonic acid be a physiological mediator of cell death?" *Cell Biochemistry and Function* 21 (2003): 97–104.

Raz I, Edor R, Cernea S, and Shafrir E. "Diabetes: insulin resistance and derangements in lipid metabolism. Cure through intervention in fat transport and storage." *Diabetes/Metabolism Research and Reviews* 21 (2005): 3–14.

Rzehak P, Meisinger C, Woelke G, Brasche S, Strube G, and Heinrich J. "Weight change, weight cycling and mortality in the ERFORT Male Cohort Study." *European Journal of Epidemiology* 22 (2007): 665–673.

Savva SC, Chadjigeorgiou C, Hatzis C, Kyriakakis M, Tsimbinos G, Tornaritis M, and Kafatos A. "Association of adipose tissue arachidonic acid content with BMI and overweight status in children from Cyprus and Crete." *British Journal of Nutrition* 91 (2004): 643–649.

Shin MJ, Hyun YJ, Kim OY, Kim JY, Jang Y, and Lee JH. "Weight loss effect on inflammation and LDL oxidation in metabolically healthy but obese (MHO) individuals: low inflammation and LDL oxidation in MHO women." *International Journal of Obesity* 30 (2006): 1529–1534.

Sinha D, Addya S, Murer E, and Boden G. "15-deoxy-delta(12, 14) prostaglandin J2: A putative endogenous promoter of adipogenesis suppresses the ob gene." *Metabolism* 48 (1999): 786–791.

Strissel KJ, Stancheva Z, Miyoshi H, Perfield JW, De Furia J, Jick Z, Greenberg AS, and Obin MS. "Adipocyte death, adipose tissue remodeling, and obesity complications." *Diabetes* 56 (2007): 2910–2918.

Taubes G. *Good Calories, Bad Calories*. New York: Alfred Knopf, 2007.

Todoric J, Löffler M, Huber J, Bilban M, Reimers M, Kadl A, Zeyda M, Waldhäusl W, and Stulnig TM. "Adipose tissue inflammation induced by high-fat diet in obese diabetic mice is prevented by n-3 polyunsaturated fatty acids." *Diabetologia* 49 (2006): 2109–2119.

Unger RH. "Longevity, lipotoxicity and leptin: the adipocyte defense against feasting and famine." *Biochimie* 87 (2005): 57–64.

———. "Weapons of lean body mass destruction: the role of ectopic lipids in the metabolic syndrome." *Endocrinology* 144 (2003): 5159–5165.

Unger RH and Zhou YT. "Lipotoxicity of beta-cells in obesity and in other causes of fatty acid spillover." *Diabetes* 50 (2001): S118–121.

Williams ES, Baylin A, and Campos H. "Adipose tissue arachidonic acid and the metabolic syndrome in Costa Rican adults." *Clinical Nutrition* 26 (2007): 474–482.

Chapter 7: Do You Have Toxic Fat Syndrome?

Boizel R, Behhamou PY, Lardy B, Laporte F, Foulon T, and Halimi S. "Ratio of triglycerides to HDL cholesterol is an indicator of LDL particle size in patients with type 2 diabetes and normal HDL cholesterol levels." *Diabetes Care* 23 (2000): 1679–1685.

Campbell B, Badrick T, Flatman R, and Kanowshi D. "Limited clinical utility of high-sensitivity plasma C-reactive protein assays." *Annals of Clinical Biochemistry* 39 (2002): 85–88.

Campbell B, Flatman R, Badrick T, and Kanowshi D. "Problems with high-sensitivity C-reactive protein." *Clinical Chemistry* 49 (2003): 201.

Crijns SA, Frummer RJ, Wichers M, Lousberg R, Clis S, and Honig A. "Altered omega-3 polyunsaturated fatty acid status in depressed post-myocardial infarction patients." *Acta Psychiatrica Scandinavica* 115 (2007): 35–40.

Danesh J, Wheeler JG, Hirschfield GM, Eiriksdottir G, Remley A, Lowe GD, Pepys MB, and Gudnason J. "C-reactive protein and other circulating markers of inflammation in the prediction of coronary heart disease." *New England Journal of Medicine* 350 (2004): 1387–1397.

Harris JI, Hibbeln JR, Mackey RH, and Muldoon MF. "Statin treatment alters serum n-3 and n-6 fatty acids in hypercholesterolemic patients." *Prostaglandins, Leukotrienes and Essential Fatty Acids* 71 (2004): 263–269.

Iso H, Sato S, Falsm AR, Shimamoto T, Terao A, Munger RG, Kitamure A, Konishi M, Iida M, and Komachi Y. "Serum fatty acids and fish intake in rural Japanese, urban Japanese, Japanese American and Caucasian American men." *International Journal of Epidemiology* 18 (1989): 374–381.

Jeppesen J, Hein HO, Suadicani P, and Gyntelberg F. "Low triglycerides-high high-density lipoprotein cholesterol and risk of ischemic heart disease." *Archives of Internal Medicine* 161 (2001): 361–366.

Kagawa Y, Nishizawa M, Suzuki M, Miyatake T, Hamamoto T, Goto K, Motonaga E, Izumikawa H, Hirata H, and Ebihara A. "Eicosapolyenoic acid of serum lipids of Japanese islanders with low incidence of cardiovascular diseases." *Journal of Nutritional Science and Vitaminology* 28 (1982): 441–453.

Lamarche B, Tchernot A, Mauriege P, Cantin B, Gagenais GR, Lupien PJ, and Despres JP. "Fasting insulin and apolipoprotein B levels and low-density particle size as risk factors for ischemic heart disease." *JAMA* 279 (1998): 1955–1961.

McLaughlin T, Abbasi F, Cheal K, Chu J, Lamendola C, and Reaven G. "Use of metabolic markers to identify overweight individuals who are insulin resistant." *Annals of Internal Medicine* 139 (2003): 802–809.

McLaughlin T, Reaven G, Abbasi F, Lamendola C, Saad M, Waters D, Simon J, and Krauss RM. "Is there a simple way to identify insulin-resistant individuals at increased risk of cardiovascular disease?" *American Journal of Cardiology* 96 (2005): 399–404.

Nesto RW. "Beyond low-density lipoprotein: addressing the atherogenic lipid triad in type 2 diabetes mellitus and the metabolic syndrome." *American Journal of Cardiovascular Drugs* 5 (2005): 379–387.

Pedersen HS, Muvad G, Sedelin KN, Malcom GT, and Boudreau DA. "N-3 fatty acids as a risk factor for hemorrhagic stroke." *Lancet* 353 (1999): 812–813.

Sandau CD, Ayotte P, Dewailly E, Duffe J, and Norstrom RJ. "Analysis of hydroxy-lated metabolites of PCBs (OH-PCBs) and other chlorinated phenolic compounds in whole blood from Canadian Inuit." *Environmental Health Perspectives* 108 (2000): 611–616.

Sears B. *The Anti-Aging Zone.* New York: Regan Books, 1999.

———. *The Anti-Inflammation Zone.* New York: Regan Books, 2005.

———. *The OmegaRx Zone.* New York: Regan Books, 2002.

———. *The Zone.* New York: Regan Books, 1995.

Tall AR. "C-reactive protein reassessed." *New England Journal of Medicine* 350 (2004): 1450–1452.

Yamada T, Strong JP, Ishii T, Ueno T, Koyama M, Wagayama H, Shimizu A, Sakai T, Malcom GT, and Guzman MA. "Atherosclerosis and omega-3 fatty acids in the populations of a fishing village and a farming village in Japan." *Atherosclerosis* 153 (2000): 469–481.

Yeni-Komshian H, Caratoni M, Abbasi F, and Reaven GM. "Relationship between several surrogate estimates of insulin resistance and quantification of insulin-mediated glucose disposal in 490 healthy nondiabetic volunteers." *Diabetes Care* 23 (2000): 171–175.

Yokoyama M, Origasa H, Matsuzaki M, Matsuzawa Y, Saito Y, Ishikawa Y, Oikawa S, Sasaki J, Hishida H, Itakura H, Kita T, Kitabatake A, Nakaya N, Sakata T, Shimada K, and Shirato K. "Effects of eicosapentaenoic acid on major coronary events in hyper-cholesterolaemic patients (JELIS): a randomized open-label, blinded endpoint analysis." *Lancet* 369 (2007): 1090–1098.

Chapter 8: The Zone Diet: Your Primary Defense in Fighting Toxic Fat

Agus MS, Swain JF, Larson CL, Eckert EA, and Ludwig DS. "Dietary composition and physiologic adaptations to energy restriction." *American Journal of Clinical Nutrition* 71 (2000): 901–907.

Ambring A, Johansson M, Axelsen M, Gan L, Strandvik B, and Friberg P.

"Mediterranean-inspired diet lowers the ratio of serum phospholipids n-6 to n-3 fatty acids, the number of leukocytes and platelets, and vascular endothelial growth factor in healthy subjects." *American Journal of Clinical Nutrition* 83 (2006): 575–581.

Bell SJ and Sears B. "Low glycemic load diets: impact on obesity and chronic diseases." *Critical Reviews in Food Science and Nutrition* 43 (2003): 357–377.

———. "A proposal for a new national diet: a low glycemic load diet with a unique macronutrient composition." *Metabolic Syndrome and Related Disorders* 1 (2003): 199–208.

Brenner RR. "Hormonal modulation of delta-6- and delta-5-desaturases: case of diabetes." *Prostaglandins, Leukotrienes and Essential Fatty Acids* 68 (2003): 151–162.

———. "Nutrition and hormonal factors influencing desaturation of essential fatty acids." *Progress in Lipid Research* 20 (1982): 41–48.

Collier G and Johnson DR. "The paradox of satiation." *Physiology and Behavior* 82 (2004): 149–153.

Dumesnil JG, Turgeon J, Tremblay A, Poirier P, Gilbert M, Gagnon L, St-Pierre S, Garneau C, Lemieux I, Pascot A, Bergeron J, and Despres JP. "Effect of a low-glycaemic index—low-fat—high protein diet on the atherogenic metabolic risk profile of abdominally obese men." *British Journal of Nutrition* 86 (2001): 557–568.

Eaton SB and Konner MJ. "Paleolithic nutrition." *New England Journal of Medicine* 312 (1985): 283–289.

Eaton SB, Shostak M, and Konner M. *The Paleolithic Prescription.* New York: Harper and Row, 1988.

Ebbeling CB, Leidig MM, Feldman HA, Lovesky MM, and Ludwig DS. "Effects of a low-glycemic load vs. low-fat diet in obese young adults: a randomized trial." *JAMA* 297 (2007): 2092–2102.

el Boustani S, Gausse JE, Descomps B, Monnier L, Mendy F, and Crastes de Paulet A. "Direct in vivo characterization of the delta-5-desaturase activity in humans by deuterium labeling: effect of insulin." *Journal of Clinical Endocrinology and Metabolism* 38 (1989): 315–321.

Fontana L, Meyer TE, Klein S, and Holloszy JO. "Long-term calorie restriction is highly effective in reducing the risk for atherosclerosis in humans." *Proceedings of the National Academy of Sciences (USA)* 101 (2004): 6659–6663.

Fontani G, Corradeschi F, Felici A, Alfatti F, Bugarini R, Fiaschi AI, Cerretani D,

Bibliography

Montorfano G, Rizzo AM, and Berra B. "Blood profiles, body fat and mood state in healthy subjects on different diets supplemented with omega-3 polyunsaturated fatty acids." *European Journal of Clinical Investigation* 35 (2005): 499–507.

Foster GD, Wyatt HR, Hill JO, McGuckin BG, Brill C, Mohammed BS, Szapary PO, Rader DJ, Edman JS, and Klein S. "A randomized trial of a low-carbohydrate diet for obesity." *New England Journal of Medicine* 22 (2003): 2082–2090.

Gannon MC, Nuttall FQ, Saeed A, Jordan K, and Hoover H. "An increase in dietary protein improves the blood glucose response in persons with type 2 diabetes." *American Journal of Clinical Nutrition* 78 (2003): 734–741.

Jenkins DJ, Wolever TM, Taylor RH, Barker H, Fielden H, Baldwin JM, Bowling AC, Newman HC, Jenkins AL, and Goff DV. "Glycemic index of foods: a physiological basis for carbohydrate exchange." *American Journal of Clinical Nutrition* 34 (1981): 362–366.

Johnston CS, Day CS, and Swan PD. "Postprandial thermogenesis is increased 100% on a high-protein, low-fat diet versus a high-carbohydrate, low-fat diet in healthy, young women." *Journal of the American College of Nutrition* 21 (2002): 55–61.

Johnston CS, Tjonn SL, and Swan PD. "High-protein, low-fat diets are effective for weight loss and favorably alter biomarkers in healthy adults." *Journal of Nutrition* 134 (2004): 586–591.

Johnston CS, Tjonn SL, Swan PD, White A, Hutchins H, and Sears B. "Ketogenic low-carbohydrate diets have no metabolic advantage over nonketogenic low-carbohydrate diets." *American Journal of Clinical Nutrition* 83 (2006): 1055–1061.

Joslin Diabetes Research Center Dietary Guidelines, www.joslin.org/Files/Nutrition_Guideline_Graded.pdf.

Layman DK, Shiue H, Sather C, Erickson DJ, and Baum J. "Increased dietary protein modifies glucose and insulin homeostasis in adult women during weight loss." *Journal of Nutrition* 133 (2003): 405–410.

Layman DK, Boileau RA, Erickson DJ, Painter JE, Shiue H, Sather C, and Christou DD. "A reduced ratio of dietary carbohydrate to protein improves body composition and blood lipid profiles during weight loss in adult women." *Journal of Nutrition* 133 (2003): 411–417.

Liu S, Manson JE, Stampfer MJ, Holmes MD, Hu FB, Hankinson SE, and Willett WC. "Dietary glycemic load assessed by food-frequency questionnaire in relation to plasma high-density-lipoprotein cholesterol and fasting plasma triacylglycerols in postmenopausal women." *American Journal of Clinical Nutrition* 73 (2001): 560–566.

Liu S, Manson JE, Buring JE, Stampfer MJ, Willett WC, and Ridker PM. "Relation between a diet with a high glycemic load and plasma concentrations of high-sensitivity C-reactive protein in middle-aged women." *American Journal of Clinical Nutrition* 75 (2002): 492–498.

Liu S, Willett WC, Stampfer MJ, Hu FB, Franz M, Sampson L, Hennekens CH, and Manson JE. "A prospective study of dietary glycemic load, carbohydrate intake, and risk of coronary heart disease in US women." *American Journal of Clinical Nutrition* 71 (2002): 1455–1461.

Ludwig DS, Majzoub JA, Al-Zahrani A, Dallal GE, Blanco I, Roberts SB, Agus MS, Swain JF, Larson CL, and Eckert EA. "Dietary high glycemic index foods, overeating, and obesity." *Pediatrics* 103 (1999): E26.

Markovic TP, Campbell LV, Balasubramanian S, Jenkins AB, Fleury AC, Simons LA, and Chisholm DJ. "Beneficial effect on average lipid levels from energy restriction and fat loss in obese individuals with or without type 2 diabetes." *Diabetes Care* 21 (1998): 695–700.

Markovic TP, Jenkins AB, Campbell LV, Furler SM, Kraegen EW, and Chisholm DJ. "The determinants of glycemic responses to diet restriction and weight loss in obesity and NIDDM." *Diabetes Care* 21 (1998): 687–694.

McCullough ML, Feskanich D, Rimm EB, Giovannucci EL, Ascherio A, Variyam JN, Spegelman D, Stampfer MJ, and Willett WC. "Adherence to the dietary guidelines for Americans and the risk of major chronic disease in men." *American Journal of Clinical Nutrition* 72 (2000): 1223–1231.

McCullough ML, Feskanich D, Stampfer MJ, Rosner BA, Hu FB, Hunter DJ, Variyam JN, Colditz GA, and Willett WC. "Adherence to the dietary guidelines for Americans and risk of major chronic disease in women." *American Journal of Clinical Nutrition* 72 (2000): 1214–1222.

Mitrou PN, Kipnis V, Thiebaut AC, Reedy J, Subar AF, Wirfalt E, Flood A, Mouw T, Hollenbeck AR, Leitzmann MF, and Schatzkin A. "Mediterranean dietary pattern and prediction of all-cause mortality in a US population: results from the NIH-AARP Diet and Health Study." *Archives of Internal Medicine* 167 (2007): 2461–2468.

Murphy KG and Bloom SR. "Gut hormones and the regulation of energy homeostasis." *Nature* 444 (2006): 854–859.

Bibliography

Naslund E and Hellstrom PM. "Appetite signaling: from gut peptides and enteric nerves to brain." *Physiology and Behavior* 92 (2007): 256–262.

Nuttall FQ, Gannon MC, Saeed A, Jordan K, and Hoover H. "The metabolic response of subjects with type 2 diabetes to a high-protein, weight-maintenance diet." *Journal of Clinical Endocrinology and Metabolism* 88 (2003): 3577–3583.

Osei-Hyiaman D, Harvey-White J, Batkai S, and Kunos G. "The role of the endocannabinoid system in the control of energy homeostasis." *International Journal of Obesity* 30 (2006): S33–38.

Pagotto U and Pasquali R. "Fighting obesity and associated risk factors by antagonizing cannabinoid type 1 receptors." *Lancet* 365 (2005): 1363–1364.

Pagotto U, Marsicano G, Cota D, Lutz B, and Pasquali R. "The emerging role of the endocannabinoid system in endocrine regulation and energy balance." *Endocrine Reviews* 27 (2006): 73–100.

Pelikonova T, Kohout M, Base J, Stefka Z, Kovar L, Kerdova L, and Valek J. "Effect of acute hyperinsulinemia on fatty acid composition of serum lipid in non-insulin dependent diabetics and healthy men." *Clinica Chimica Acta* 203 (1991): 329–337.

Pereira MA, Swain J, Goldfine AB, Rifai N, and Ludwig DS. "Effects of a low-glycemic load diet on resting energy expenditure and heart disease risk factors during weight loss." *JAMA* 292 (2004): 2482–2490.

Pittas AG, Roberts SB, Das SK, Gilhooly CH, Saltzman E, Golden J, Stark PC, and Greenberg AS. "The effects of the dietary glycemic load on type 2 diabetes risk factors during weight loss." *Obesity* 14 (2006): 2200–2209.

Pittas AG, Das SK, Hajduk CL, Golden J, Saltzman E, Stark PC, Greenberg AS, and Roberts SB. "A low-glycemic load diet facilitates greater weight loss in overweight adults with high insulin secretion but not in overweight adults with low insulin secretion in the CALERIE Trial." *Diabetes Care* 28 (2005): 2939–2941.

Sears B. *Mastering the Zone*. New York: Regan Books, 1997.

———. *The Anti-Inflammation Zone*. New York: Regan Books, 2005.

———. *The OmegaRx Zone*. New York: Regan Books, 2002.

———. *The Zone*. New York: Regan Books, 1995.

———. *Zone Perfect Meals*. New York: Regan Books, 1998.

Sears B and Bell SJ. "The Zone Diet: an anti-inflammatory, low glycemic-load diet." *Metabolic Syndrome and Related Disorders* 2 (2004): 24–38.

Sears B and Sears L. *Zone Meals in Seconds.* New York: Regan Books, 2001.

Silver MJ, Hoch W, Kocsis JJ, Ingerman CM, and Smith JB. "Arachidonic acid causes sudden death in rabbits." *Science* 183 (1974): 1085–1087.

Skov AR, Toubro S, Ronn B, Holm L, and Astrup A. "Randomized trial on protein vs carbohydrate in ad libitum fat reduced diet for the treatment of obesity." *International Journal of Obesity and Related Metabolic Disorders* 23 (1999): 528–536.

Unger RH. "Glucagon and the insulin-glucagon ratio in diabetes and other catabolic illnesses." *Diabetes* 20 (1971): 834–838.

Unger RH and Lefebvre PJ. *Glucagon: Molecular Physiology, Clinical and Therapeutic Implications.* Oxford: Pergamon Press, 1972.

Whitten P. "Stanford's Secret Weapon." *Swimming World* (1993).

Wolfe BM and Piche LA. "Replacement of carbohydrate by protein in a conventional-fat diet reduces cholesterol and triglyceride concentrations in healthy normolipidemic subjects." *Clinical and Investigative Medicine* 22 (1999): 140–148.

Chapter 9: Super Fish Oil: Your Final Defense in Fighting Toxic Fat

Arisawa K, Matsummura T, Tohyama C, Saito H, Satoh H, Hagai M, Morita M, and Suzuki T. "Fish intake, plasma omega-3 polyunsaturated fatty acids, and poly-chlorinated debenzo-p-dioxins/polychlorinated dibenzo-furans and co-planar polychlorinated biphenyls in the blood of the Japanese population." *International Archives of Occupational and Environmental Health* 76 (2003): 205–215.

Chavali SR and Forse RA. "Decreased production of interleukin-6 and prostaglandin E2 associated with inhibition of delta-5 desaturation of omega-6 fatty acids in mice fed safflower oil diets supplemented with sesamol." *Prostaglandins, Leukotrienes and Essential Fatty Acids* 61 (1999): 347–352.

Iso H, Sato S, Falsm AR, Shimamoto T, Terao A, Munger RG, Kitamure A, Konishi M, Iida M, and Komachi Y. "Serum fatty acids and fish intake in rual Japanese, urban Japanese, Japanese American and Caucasian American men." *International Journal of Epidemiology* 18 (1989): 374–381.

Jeng KCG and Hou RCW. "Sesamin and sesamolin: Nature's therapeutic lignans." *Current Enzyme Inhibition* 1 (2005): 11–20.

Bibliography

Kagawa Y, Nishizawa M, Suzuki M, Miyatake T, Hamamoto T, Goto K, Motonaga E, Izumikawa H, Hirata H, and Ebihara A. "Eicosapolyenoic acid of serum lipids of Japanese islanders with low incidence of cardiovascular diseases." *Journal of Nutritinal Science and Vitaminology* 28 (1982): 441–453.

Laidlaw M and Holub BJ. "Effects of supplementation with fish oil-derived n-3 fatty acids and gamma-linolenic acid on circulating plasma lipids and fatty acid profiles in women." *American Journal of Clinical Nutrition* 77 (2003): 37–42.

Nakamura T, Azuma A, Kuribayashi T, Sugihara H, Okuda S, and Nakagawa M. "Serum fatty acid levels, dietary style and coronary heart in three neighbouring areas in Japan." *British Journal of Nutrition* 89 (2003): 267–272.

Pedesen HS, Mulvad G, Seidelin KN, Malcom GT, and Doudreau DA. "N-3 fatty acids as a risk marker for haemorrhagic stroke." *Lancet* 353 (1999): 812–813.

Phinney S. "Potential risk of prolonged gamma-linolenic acid use." *Annals of Internal Medicine* 120 (1994): 692.

Sears B. *The Anti-Inflammation Zone.* New York: Regan Books, 2005.

———. *The OmegaRx Zone.* New York: Regan Books, 2002.

———. *The Zone.* New York: Regan Books, 1995.

Shimizu S, Akimoto K, Shinmen Y, Kawashima H, Sugano M, and Yamada H. "Sesamin is a potent and specific inhibitor of delta-5-desaturase in polyunsaturated fatty acid biosynthesis." *Lipids* 26 (1991): 512–516.

Sorgi PJ, Hallowell EM, Hutchins HL, and Sears B. "Effects of an open-label pilot study with high-dose EPA/DHA concentrates on plasma phospholipids and behavior in children with attention deficit hyperactivity disorder." *Nutrition Journal* 6 (2007): 16.

Yamada T, Strong JP, Ishii T, Ueno T, Koyama M, Wagayama H, Shimizu A, Sakai T, Malcom GT, and Guzman MA. "Atherosclerosis and omega-3 fatty acids in the populations of fishing village and a farming village in Japan." *Atherosclerosis* 153 (2000): 469–481.

Yokoyama M, Origasa H, Matsuzaki M, Matsuzawa Y, Saito Y, Ishikawa Y, Oikawa S, Sasaki J, Hishida H, Itakura H, Kita T, Kitabatake A, Nakaya N, Sakata T, Shimada K, and Shirato K. "Effects of eicosapentaenoic acid on major coronary events in hypercholesterolaemic patients (JELIS): a randomized open-label, blinded endpoint analysis." *Lancet* 369 (2007): 1090–1098.

Zuijdgeest-van Leeuwen SD, Dagnelie PC, Rietveld T, van den Berg JWO, and Wilson JHP. "Incorporation and washout of orally administered n-3 fatty acid ethyl esters in different plasma lipid fractions." *International Archives of Occupational and Environmental Health* 82 (1999): 481–488.

Chapter 10: Putting It All Together

Biesalski HK. "Polyphenols and inflammation: basic interactions." *Current Opinion in Clinical Nutrition and Metabolic Care* 10 (2007): 724–728.

Gluckman P and Hanson M. *Mismatch.* New York: Oxford University Press, 2006.

Scalbert A, Johnson IT, and Saltmarsh M. "Polyphenols: antioxidants and beyond." *American Journal of Clinical Nutrition* 81 (2005): 215S–217S.

Sears B. *A Week in the Zone.* New York: Regan Books, 2000.

———. *Mastering the Zone.* New York: Regan Books, 1997.

———. *The Anti-Inflammation Zone.* New York: Regan Books, 2005.

———. *The Zone.* New York: Regan Books, 1995.

———. *What to Eat in the Zone.* New York: Regan Books, 2003.

———. *Zone Food Blocks.* New York: Regan Books, 1998.

———. *Zone Perfect Meals in Minutes.* New York: Regan Books, 1997.

Sears B and Sears L. *Zone Meals in Seconds.* New York: Regan Books, 2004.

Yoon JH and Baek SJ. "Molecular targets of dietary polyphenols with anti-inflammatory properties." *Yonsei Medical Journal* 46 (2005): 585–596.

Chapter 11: Overcoming Obstacles to Your Success

Avena NM, Long KA, and Hoebel BG. "Sugar-dependent rats show enhanced responding for sugar after abstinence: evidence of a sugar deprivation effect." *Physiology and Behavior* 84 (2005): 359–362.

Banks WA, Coon AB, Robinson SM, Moinuddin A, Shultz JM, Nakaoke R, and Morley JE. "Triglycerides induce leptin resistance at the blood-brain barrier." *Diabetes* 53 (2004): 1253–1260.

Chen K, Li F, Li J, Cai H, Strom S, Bisello A, Kelley DE, Friedman-Einat M, Skibinski GA, McCrory MA, Szalai AJ, and Zhao AZ. "Induction of leptin resistance through direct interaction of C-reactive protein with leptin." *Nature Medicine* 12 (2006): 425–432.

Colantuoni C, Schwenker J, McCarthy J, Rada P, Ladenheim B, Cadet JL, Schwartz GJ, Moran TH, and Hoebel BG. "Excessive sugar intake alters binding to dopamine and mu-opioid receptors in the brain." *NeuroReport* 12 (2001): 3549–3552.

Darmon N, Darmon M, Maillot M, and Drewnowski A. "A nutrient density standard for vegetables and fruits: nutrients per calorie and nutrients per unit cost." *Journal of the American Dietetic Association* 105 (2005): 1881–1887.

Despres JP, Golay A, and Sjostrom L. "Effects of rimonabant on metabolic risk factors in overweight patients with dyslipidemia." *New England Journal of Medicine* 353 (2005): 2121–2134.

Drewnowski A and Specter SE. "Poverty and obesity: the role of energy density and energy costs." *American Journal of Clinical Nutrition* 79 (2004): 6–16.

Drewnowski A, Darmon N, and Briend A. "Replacing fats and sweets with vegetables and fruits—a question of cost." *American Journal of Public Health* 94 (2004): 1555–1559.

Enriori PJ, Evans AE, Sinnayah P, and Cowley MA. "Leptin resistance and obesity." *Obesity* 14 Suppl 5 (2006): 254S–258S.

Grossman E. "Chemicals may play role in rise of obesity." *Washington Post*, March 12, 2007, A06.

Grun F, Watanabe H, Zamanian Z, Maeda L, Arima K, Cubacha R, Gardiner DM, Kanno J, Iguchi T, and Blumberg B. "Endocrine-disrupting organotin compounds are potent inducers of adipogenesis in vertebrates." *Molecular Endocrinology* 20 (2006): 2141–2155.

Heindel JJ. "Endocrine disruptors and the obesity epidemic." *Toxicological Sciences* 76 (2003): 247–249.

Keith SW, Redden DT, Katzmarzyk PT, Boggiano MM, Hanlon EC, Benca RM, Ruden D, Pietrobelli A, Barger JL, Kontaine KR, Wang C, Aronne LJ, Wright SM, Baskin M, Dhurandhar NV, Lijoi MC, Grilo CM, DeLuca M, Westfall AO, and Allison DB. "Putative contributors to the secular increase in obesity: exploring the roads less traveled." *International Journal of Obesity* 30 (2006): 1585–1594.

Knutson KL, Spiegel K, Penev P, and Van Cauter E. "The metabolic consequences of sleep deprivation." *Sleep Medicine Reviews* 11 (2007): 163–178.

Kolata G. *Rethinking Thin*. New York: Farrar, Straus, and Giroux, 2006.

Lenoir M, Serre F, Cantin L, and Ahmed SH. "Intense sweetness surpasses cocaine reward." *PLoS ONE 2* (2007): e698.

Masumo H, Kidani T, Sekiya K, Saykama K, Shiosaka T, Yamamoto H, and Honda K. "Bisphenol A in combination with insulin can accelerate the conversion of 3T3L1 fibroblasts to adipocytes." *Journal of Lipid Research* 43 (2002): 676–684.

Miller WC, Koceja DM, and Hamilton EJ. "A meta-analysis of the past 25 years of weight loss research using diet, exercise or diet plus exercise intervention." *International Journal of Obesity and Related Metabolic Disorders* 21 (1997): 941–947.

Monsivais P and Drewnowski A. "The rising cost of low-energy-density foods." *Journal of the American Dietetic Association* 107 (2007): 2071–2076.

Naska A, Oikonomou E, Trichopoulou A, Psaltopoulou T, and Trichopoulos D. "Siesta in healthy adults and coronary mortality in the general population." *Archives of Internal Medicine* 167 (2007): 296–301.

Nestle M. *Food Politics*. Berkeley: University of California Press, 2002.

———. *What to Eat*. New York: North Point Press, 2006.

Oda E. "n-3 fatty acids and the endocannabinoid system." *American Journal of Clinical Nutrition* 85 (2007): 919.

Pollan M. *The Omnivore's Dilemma*. New York: Penguin Press, 2006.

Rosenbaum M, Goldsmith R, Bloomfield D, Magnano A, Weimer L, Heymsfield S, Gallagher D, Mayer L, Murphy E, and Leibel RL. "Low-dose leptin reverses skeletal muscle, autonomic, and neuroendocrine adaptations to maintenance of reduced weight." *Journal of Clinical Investigation* 115 (2005): 3579–3586.

Sakurai K, Kawazuma M, Adachi T, Harigaya T, Saito Y, Hashimoto N, and Mori C. "Bisphenol A affects glucose transport in mouse 3T3-F442A adipocytes." *British Journal of Pharmacology* 141 (2004): 209–214.

Sears B. *The Anti-Aging Zone*. New York: Regan Books, 1999.

Spangler R, Wittkowski KM, Goddard NL, Avena NM, Hoebel BG, and Leibowitz SF. "Opiate-like effects of sugar on gene expression in reward areas of the rat brain." *Brain Research Molecular Brain Research* 124 (2004): 134–142.

Spiegel K, Knutson K, Leproult R, Tasali E, and Van Cauter E. "Sleep loss: a novel risk factor for insulin resistance and Type 2 diabetes." *Journal of Applied Physiology* 99 (2005): 2008–2019.

Taubes G. *Good Calories, Bad Calories.* New York: Alfred Knopf, 2007.

Watanabe S, Doshi M, and Hamazakibi T. "n-3 polyunsaturated fatty acid (PUFA) deficiency elevates and n-3 PUFA enrichment reduces brain 2-arachidonylglycerol level in mice." *Prostaglandins, Leukotrienes and Essential Fatty Acids* 69 (2003): 51–59.

Chapter 12: The Coming Reckoning

Cauchon D. "Bill for taxpayers swells by trillions." *USA Today*, May 19, 2008.

Lawlor EF. *Redesigning the Medicare Contract.* Chicago: University of Chicago Press, 2003.

Kotlifoff LJ. *The Healthcare Fix.* Cambridge: MIT Press, 2007.

Marmor TR. *The Politics of Medicare.* New York: Aldine de Gruyter, 2000.

Nestle M. *Food Politics.* Berkeley: University of California Press, 2002.

Olshansky SJ, Passaro DJ, Hershow RC, Layden J, Carnes BA, Brody J, Hayflick L, Butler RN, Allison DB, and Ludwig DS. "A potential decline in life expectancy in the United States in the 21st century." *New England Journal of Medicine* 352 (2005): 1138–1145.

Saviro D. *Who Should Pay for Medicare?* Chicago: University of Chicago Press, 2004.

Appendix C—Hormones: The Keys to Your Biological Internet

Arora S. "The role of neuropeptides in appetite regulation and obesity." *Neuropeptides* 40 (2006): 375–401.

Balcioglu A and Wurtman RJ. "Effects of fenfluramine and phentermine (fen–phen) on dopamine and serotonin release in rat striatum: in vivo microdialysis study in conscious animals." *Brain Research* 813 (1998): 67–72.

Bloom SR, Wayne K, and Chaudhri O. "Gut feeling—the secret of satiety?" *Clinical Medicine* 5 (2005): 147–152.

Burton-Freeman B, Davis PA, and Schneeman BO. "Plasma cholecystolkinin is associated with subjective measures of satiety in women." *American Journal of Clinical Nutrition* 76 (2002): 659–667.

Chan JL, Mun EC, Stoyneva V, Mantzoros CS, and Goldfine AB. "Peptide YY levels are elevated after gastric bypass surgery." *Obesity* 14 (2006): 194–198.

de Graff C, Blom W, Smeets P, Stafleu A, and Hendriks HF. "Biomarkers of satiation and satiety." *American Journal of Clinical Nutrition* 79 (2004): 946–961.

Itoh M, Suganami T, Satoh N, Tanimoto-Koyama K, Yuan X, Tanaka M, Kawano H, Yano T, Aoe S, Takeya M, Shimatsu A, Kuzuya H, Kamei Y, and Ogawa Y. "Increased adiponectin secretion by highly purified eicosapentaenoic acid in rodent models of obesity and human obese subjects." *Arteriosclerosis, Thrombosis, and Vascular Biology* 27 (2007): 1918–1925.

Korner J, Inabnet W, Conwell IM, Taveras C, Daud A, Olivero-Rivera L, Restuccia NL, and Bessler M. "Differential effects of gastric bypass and banding on circulating gut hormone and leptin levels." *Obesity* 14 (2006): 1553–1561.

le Roux CW, Welbourn R, Werling M, Osborne A, Kokkinos A, Laurenius A, Lonroth H, Fandriks L, Ghatei MA, Bloom SR, and Olbers T. "Gut hormones as mediators of appetite and weight loss after Roux-en-Y gastric bypass." *Annals of Surgery* 246 (2007): 780–785.

Matzinger D, Gutzwiller J, Drewe J, Orban A, Engel R, D'Amato M, Rovati L, and Beglinger C. "Inhibition of food intake in response to intestinal lipids is mediated by cholecystolkinin in humans." *American Journal of Physiology* 277 (1999): R1718–1724.

Murphy KC and Bloom SR. "Gut hormones in the control of appetite." *Experimental Physiology* 89 (2004): 507–516.

Neary NM, Goldstone AP, and Bloom SR. "Appetite regulation: From the gut to the hypothalamus." *Clinical Endocrinology* 60 (2003): 153–160.

Neschen S, Morino K, Rossbacher JC, Pongratz RL, Cline GW, Sono S, Gillum M, and Shulman GI. "Fish oil regulates adiponectin secretion by a peroxisome proliferator-activated receptor gamma-dependent mechanism in mice." *Diabetes* 55 (2006): 924–928.

Oda E. "n-3 fatty acids and the endocannabinoid system." *American Journal of Clinical Nutrition* 85 (2007): 919.

Osei-Hyiaman D, Harvey-White J, Batkai S, and Kunos G. "The role of the endocannabinoid system in the control of energy homeostasis." *International Journal of Obesity* 30 (2006): S33–38.

Sears B. *The Anti-Aging Zone.* New York: Regan Books, 1999.

Bibliography

———. *The Zone.* New York: Regan Books, 1995.

Watanabe S, Doshi M, and Hamazaki T. "n-3 polyunsaturated fatty acid (PUFA) deficiency elevates and n-3 PUFA enrichment reduces brain 2-arachidonylglycerol level in mice." *Prostaglandins, Leukotrienes and Essential Fatty Acids* 69 (2003): 51–59.

Appendix D—Eicosanoids: Hormones of Mystery

Ankel H, Turriziani O, and Antonelli G. "Prostaglandin A inhibits replication of human immunodeficiency virus during acute infection." *Journal of General Virology* 72 (1991): 2797–2800.

Bourre JM, Piciotti M, and Dumont O. "Delta-6-desaturase in brain and liver during development and aging." *Lipids* 25 (1990): 354–356.

Brenner RR. "Nutrition and hormonal factors influencing desaturation of essential fatty acids." *Progress in Lipid Research* 20 (1982): 41–48.

Burr GO and Burr MR. "A new deficiency disease produced by rigid exclusion of fat from the diet." *Journal of Biological Chemistry* 82 (1929): 345–367.

Chapkin RS, Somer SD, and Erickson KL. "Dietary manipulation of macrophage phospholipids classes: selective increase in dihomo gamma linolenic acid." *Lipids* 23 (1988): 766–770.

Chavali SR and Forse RA. "Decreased production of interleukin-6 and prostaglandin E2 associated with inhibition of delta-5-desaturation of omega 6 fatty acids in mice fed safflower oil diets supplemented with sesamol." *Prostaglandins, Leukotrienes and Essential Fatty Acids* 61 (1999): 347–352.

Cho HP, Nakamura M, and Clarke SD. "Cloning, expression, and fatty acid regulation of human delta-5-desaturase." *Journal of Biological Chemistry* 274 (1999): 37335–37399.

Clarke SD. "Polyunsaturated fatty acid regulation of gene transcription: a mechanism to improve energy balance and insulin resistance." *British Journal of Nutrition* 83 (2000): S59–S66.

Conquer JA and Holub BJ. "Dietary docosahexaenoic acid as a source of eicosapentaenoic acid in vegetarians and omnivores." *Lipids* 32 (1997): 341–345.

el Boustani S, Gausse JE, Descomps B, Monnier L, Mendy F, and Crastes de Paulet A. "Direct in vivo characterization of the delta-5-desaturase activity in humans by deuterium labeling: effect of insulin." *Journal of Clinical Endocrinology and Metabolism* 38 (1989): 315–321.

Ferreria SH, Moncada S, and Vane JR. "Indomethacin and aspirin abolish prostaglandin release from the spleen." *Nature New Biology* 231 (1971): 237–239.

Garg ML, Thomson ABR, and Clandinin MT. "Effect of dietary cholesterol and/or omega-3 fatty acids on lipid composition and delta-5-desaturase activity of rat liver microsomes." *Journal of Nutrition* 118 (1998): 661–668.

Hill EG, Johnson SB, Lawson LD, Mahfouz MM, and Holman RT. "Perturbation of the metabolism of essential fatty acids by dietary partially hydrogenated vegetable oil." *Proceedings of the National Academy of Sciences (USA)* 79 (1982): 953–957.

Jensen RG, Ferris AM, and Lammi-Keefe CJ. "Lipids in human milk and infant formulas." *Annual Review of Nutrition* 12 (1992): 417–441.

Laidlaw M and Holub BJ. "Effects of supplementation with fish oil-derived n-3 fatty acids and gamma-linolenic acid on circulating plasma lipids and fatty acid profiles in women." *American Journal of Clinical Nutrition* 77 (2003): 37–42.

Levy BD. "Myocardial 15-epi-lipoxin A4 generation provides a new mechanism for the immunomodulatory effects of statins and thiazolidinediones." *Circulation* 114 (2006): 873–875.

Oates JA. "The 1982 Nobel prize in physiology or medicine." *Science* 218 (1982): 765–768.

Pelikonova T, Kohout M, Base J, Stefka Z, Kovar L, Kerdova L, and Valek J. "Effect of acute hyperinsulinemia on fatty acid composition of serum lipid in non-insulin dependent diabetics and healthy men." *Clinica Chimica Acta* 203 (1991): 329–337.

Phinney S. "Potential risk of prolonged gamma-linolenic acid use." *Annals Internal Medicine* 120 (1994): 692.

Plourde M and Cunnane SC. "Extremely limited synthesis of long chain polyunsaturates in adults: implications for their dietary essentiality and use as supplements." *Applied Physiology, Nutrition, and Metabolism* 32 (2007): 619–634.

Rozera C, Carattoli A, De Marco A, Amici C, Giorgi C, and Santoro MG. "Inhibition of HIV-1 replication by cyclopentenone prostaglandins in acutely infected human cells. Evidence for a transcriptional block." *Journal of Clinical Investigation* 97 (1996): 1795–1803.

Sears B. *The Anti-Aging Zone.* New York: Regan Books, 1999.

———. *The Anti-Inflammation Zone.* New York: Regan Books, 2005.

Bibliography

————. *The OmegaRx Zone*. New York: Regan Books, 2002.

————. *The Zone*. New York: Regan Books, 1995.

Serhan CN. "Lipoxins and aspirin-triggered 15-epi-lipoxin biosynthesis: an update and role in anti-inflammation and pro-resolution." *Prostaglandins and Other Lipid Mediators* 69 (2002): 433–455.

————. "Resolution phase of inflammation: novel endogenous anti-inflammatory and proresolving lipid mediators and pathways." *Annual Review of Immunology* 25 (2007): 101–137.

Serhan CN, Arita M, Hong S, and Gotlinger K. "Resolvins, docosatrienes, and neuroprotectins, novel omega-3-derived mediators, and their endogenous aspirin-triggered epimers." *Lipids* 39 (2004): 1125–1132.

Smith DL, Willis AL, Nguyen N, Conner D, Zahedi S, and Fulks J. "Eskimo plasma constituents, dihomo gamma linolenic acid, eicosapentaenoic acid, and docosahexaenoic acid inhibit the release of atherogenic mitogens." *Lipids* 24 (1989): 70–75.

Stone KJ, Willis AL, Hurt M, Kirtland SJ, Kernof PBA, and McNichol GF. "The metabolism of dihomo gamma linolenic acid in man." *Lipids* 14 (1979): 174–180.

Trowbridge HO and Emling RC. *Inflammation. A Review of the Process—5ᵗʰ Edition*. Chicago: Quintessence Books, 1997.

Vadas P, Pruzanski W, Stefanski E, Ruse J, Farewell V, McLaughlin J, and Bombardier C. "Concordance of endogenous cortisol and phospholipase A2 levels in gram-negative septic shock: a prospective study." *Journal of Laboratory and Clinical Medicine* 111 (1998): 584–590.

Vane JR. "Inhibition of prostaglandin synthesis as a mechanism of action for aspirin-like drugs." *Nature New Biology* 231 (1971): 232–235.

Vang K and Ziboh VA. "15-lipoxygenase metabolites of gamma-linolenic acid/eicosapentaenoic acid suppress growth and arachidonic acid metabolism in human prostatic adenocarcinoma cells: possible implications of dietary fatty acids." *Prostaglandins, Leukotrienes and Essential Fatty Acids* 72 (2005): 363–372.

von Euler US. "On specific vasodilating and plain muscle stimulating substances from accessory genital glands in men and certain animals (prostaglandins and vesiglandin)." *Journal of Physiology* 88 (1936): 213–234.

Willis AL. *Handbook of Eicosanoids, Prostaglandins, and Related Lipids*. Boca Raton: CRC Press, 1987.

Appendix E—Everything You Ever Wanted to Know About Fish Oil But Were Afraid to Ask

Arisawa K, Matsumura T, Tohyama C, Saito H, Satoh H, Nagai M, Morita M, and Suzuki T. "Fish intake, plasma omega-3 polyunsaturated fatty acids, and polychlorinated dibenzo-p-dioxins/polychlorinated dibenzo-furans and co-planar polychlorinated biphenyls in the blood of the Japanese population." *International Archives of Occupational and Environmental Health* 76 (2003): 205–215.

Guy RA. "The history of cod-liver oil as a remedy." *American Journal of Diseases of Children* 26 (1923): 112–116.

Kawai K, Matsuno K, and Kasai H. "Detection of 4-oxo-2-hexenal, a novel mutagenic product of lipid peroxidation, in human diet and cooking vapor." *Mutation Research* 603 (2006): 186–192.

Mandal AK, Zhang Z, Kim S-J, Tsai P-C, and Mukherjee AB. "Ying-Yang: Balancing act of prostaglandins with opposing function to regulate inflammation." *Journal of Immunology* 175 (2005): 6271–6273.

Plourde M and Cunnane SC. "Extremely limited synthesis of long chain polyunsaturates in adults: implications for their dietary essentiality and use as supplements." *Applied Physiology, Nutrition, and Metabolism* 32 (2007): 619–634.

Rajakumar K. "Vitamin D, cod-liver oil, sunlight, and rickets: a historical perspective." *Pediatrics* 112 (2003): 132–135.

Sears B. *The Anti-Inflammation Zone.* New York: Regan Books, 2005.

———. *The OmegaRx Zone.* New York: Regan Books, 2002.

Serhan CN. "Novel omega-3 derived local mediators in anti-inflammation and resolution." *Pharmacology and Therapeutics* 105 (2005): 7–21.

Shirai N, Hayashi K, Suzuki H, and Shimizu R. "The effects of Erabu sea snake oil on the plasma lipids and glucose, and liver lipids in mice." *Nutrition Research* 22 (2002): 1197–1207.

Shirai N, Suzuki H, and Shimizu R. "Effect of Erabu sea snake Laticauda semifasciata oil intake on maze-learning ability in mice." *Fisheries Resolution* 70 (2004): 314–318.

Appendix F—Insulin Resistance: It All Starts in Your Adipose Tissue

Bays H, Mandarino H, and DeFronzo RA. "Role of the adipocyte, free fatty acids, and ectopic fat in pathogenesis of type 2 diabetes mellitus: peroxisomal proliferator-activated receptor agonists provide a rational therapeutic approach." *Journal of Clinical Endocrinology and Metabolism* 89 (2004): 463–478.

Birnbaum Y, Ye Y, Lin Y, Freeberg SY, Nishi SP, Martinez JD, Huang MH, Uretsky BF, and Perez-Polo JR. "Augmentation of myocardial production of 15-epi-lipoxin-A4 by pioglitazone and atorvastatin in the rat." *Circulation* 114 (2006): 929–935.

Blacklock CJ, Lawrence JR, Wiles D, Malcolm EA, Gibson IH, Kelly CJ, and Paterson JR. "Salicylic acid in the serum of subjects not taking aspirin. Comparison of salicylic acid concentrates in the serum of vegetarians, non-vegetarians, and patients taking low dose aspirin." *Journal of Clinical Pathology* 54 (2001): 553–555.

Bogacka I, Xie H, Bray GA, and Smith SR. "The effect of pioglitazone on peroxisome proliferator-activated receptor-gamma target genes related to lipid storage in vivo." *Diabetes Care* 27(7) (2004): 1660–1667.

Bonen A, Tandon NN, Glatz JFC, Luiken JJFP, and Heigenhauser GJF. "The fatty acid transporter FAT/CD36 is upregulated in subcutaneous and visceral adipose tissues in human obesity and type 2 diabetes." *International Journal of Obesity* 30 (2006): 877–883.

Booth GL, Kapral MK, Fung K, and Tu JV. "Relation between age and cardiovascular disease in men and women with diabetes compared with non-diabetic people." *Lancet* 368 (2006): 29–36.

Borkman M, Storlien LH, Pan DA, Jenkins AB, Chisholm DJ, and Campbell LV. "The relation between insulin sensitivity and the fatty-acid composition of skeletal-muscle phopholipids." *New England Journal of Medicine* 328 (1993): 911–917.

Borst SE. "The role of TNF-alpha in insulin resistance." *Endocrine* 23 (2004): 177–182.

Cinti S, Mitchell G, Barbatelli G, Murano I, Ceresi E, Faloia E, Wang S, Fortier M, Greenberg AS, and Obin MS. "Adipocyte death defines macrophage localization and function in adipose tissue of obese mice and humans." *Journal of Lipid Research* 46 (2005): 2347–2355.

D'Acquisto F and Ianaro A. "From willow bark to peptides: the ever widening spectrum of NF-kappaB inhibitors." *Current Opinion in Pharmacology* 6 (2006): 387–392.

Flachs P, Horakova O, Brauner P, Rossmeisl M, Pecina P, Franssen-van Hal N, Ruzickova J, Sponarova J, Drahota Z, Vlcek C, Keijer J, Houstek J, and Kopecky J.

"Polyunsaturated fatty acids of marine origin upregulate mitochondrial biogenesis and induce beta-oxidation in white fat." *Diabetologia* 48 (2005): 2365–2375.

Freeth A, Udupi V, Basile R, and Green A. "Prolonged treatment with prostaglandin E1 increases the rate of lipolysis in rat adipocytes." *Life Sciences* 73 (2003): 393–401.

Gregor MF and Hotamisligil GS. "Adipocyte stress: The endoplasmic reticulum and metabolic disease." *Journal of Lipid Research* 48 (2007): 1905–1914.

Hotamisligil GS. "Inflammation and metabolic disorders." *Nature* 444 (2006): 860–867.

Hotamisligil GS, Arner P, Caro JF, Atkinson RL, and Spiegelman BM. "Increased adipose tissue expression of tumor necrosis factor-alpha in human obesity and insulin resistance." *Journal of Clinical Investigation* 95 (1995): 2409–2415.

Huber J, Loffler M, Bilban M, Reimers M, Kadl A, Todoric J, Zeyda M, Geyeregger R, Schreiner M, Weichhart T, Leitinger N, Waldhausl W, and Stulnig TM. "Prevention of high-fat diet-induced adipose tissue remodeling in obese diabetic mice by n-3 polyunsaturated fatty acids." *International Journal of Obesity* 31 (2007): 1004–1013.

Itoh M, Suganami T, Satoh N, Tanimoto-Koyama K, Yuan X, Tanaka M, Kawano H, Yano T, Aoe S, Takeya M, Shimatsu A, Kuzuya H, Kamei Y, and Ogawa Y. "Increased adiponectin secretion by highly purified eicosapentaenoic acid in rodent models of obesity and human obese subjects." *Arteriosclerosis, Thrombosis, and Vascular Biology* 27 (2007): 1918–1925.

Kahn S, Hull RL, and Utzschneider KM. "Mechanisms linking obesity to insulin resistance and type 2 diabetes." *Nature* 444 (2007): 840–846.

Kim JK, Gimeno RE, Higashimori T, Kim H-J, Choi M, Punreddy S, Mozell RL, Tan G, Stricker-Krongrad A, Hirsch DJ, Fillmore JJ, Liu ZX, Dong J, Cline G, Stahl A, Lodish HF, and Shulman GI. "Inactivation of fatty acid transport protein 1 prevents fat-induced insulin resistance in skeletal muscle." *Journal of Clinical Investigation* 113 (2004): 756–763.

Kim JY, van de Wall E, Laplante M, Azzara A, Trujillo ME, Hofmann SM, Schraw T, Durand JL, Li H, Li G, Jelicks LA, Mehler MF, Hui DY, Deshaies Y, Shulman GI, Schwartz GJ, and Scherer PE. "Obesity-associated improvements in metabolic profile through expansion of adipose tissue." *Journal of Clinical Investigation* 117 (2007): 2621–2637.

Kiss K, Kiss J, Rudolf E, Cervinka M, and Szeberenyi J. "Sodium salicylate inhibits

Bibliography

NF-kappaB and induces apoptosis in PC12 cells." *Journal of Biochemical and Biophysical Methods* 61 (2004): 229–240.

Lehrke M and Lazar MA. "Inflamed about obesity." *Nature Medicine* 10 (2004): 126–127.

Li H, Ruan XZ, Powis SH, Fernando R, Mon WY, Wheeler DC, Moorhead JF, and Varghese Z. "EPA and DHA reduce LPS-induced inflammation responses in HK-2 cells: evidence for a PPAR-gamma-dependent mechanism." *Kidney International* 67 (2005): 867–874.

Lindmark S, Buren J, and Eriksson JW. "Insulin resistance, endocrine function and adipokines in type 2 diabetes patients at different glycaemic levels: potential impact for glucotoxicity in vivo." *Clinical Endocrinology* 65 (2006): 301–309.

Maeda K, Cao H, Kono K, Gorgun CZ, Furuhashi M, Uysal KT, Cao Q, Atsumi G, Malone H, Krishnan B, Minokoshi Y, Kahn BB, Parker RA, and Hotamisligil GS. "Adipocyte/macrophage fatty acid binding proteins control integrated metabolic responses in obesity and diabetes." *Cell Metabolism* 1 (2005): 107–119.

Maeda K, Uysal KT, Makowski L, Gorgun CZ, Atsumi G, Parker RA, Bruning J, Hertzel AV, Bernlohr DA, and Hotamisligil GS. "Role of the fatty acid binding protein mal1 in obesity and insulin resistance." *Diabetes* 52 (2003): 300–307.

Makowski L and Hotamisligil GS. "The role of fatty acid binding proteins in metabolic syndrome and atherosclerosis." *Current Opinion in Lipidology* 16 (2005): 543–548.

Manuel DG and Schultz SE. "Health-related quality of life and health-adjusted life expectancy of people with diabetes in Ontario, Canada, 1996–1997." *Diabetes Care* 27 (2004): 407–414.

Marett A. "Molecular mechanisms of inflammation in obesity-linked insulin resistance." *International Journal of Obesity* 27 (2003): S46–S48.

Mazid MA, Chowdhury AA, Nagao K, Nishimura K, Jisaka M, Nagaya T, and Yokota K. "Endogenous 15-deoxy-delta(12, 14)-prostaglandin J(2) synthesized by adipocytes during maturation phase contributes to upregulation of fat storage." *FEBS Letters* 580 (2006): 6885–6890.

McLaughlin T, Abbasi F, Lamendola C, Liang L, Reaven G, Schaaf P, and Reaven P. "Differentiation between obesity and insulin resistance in the association with C-reactive protein." *Circulation* 106 (2002): 2908–2912.

McLaughlin T, Sherman A, Tsao P, Gonzalez O, Yee G, Lamendola C, Reaven GM, and Cushman SW. "Enhanced proportion of small adipose cells in insulin-resistant vs insulin-sensitive obese individuals implicates impaired adipogenesis." *Diabetologia* 50 (2007): 1707–1715.

Neels JG and Olefsky JM. "Inflamed fat: what starts the fire?" *Journal of Clinical Investigation* 116 (2006): 33–35.

Neschen S, Morino K, Dong J, Wang-Fischer Y, Cline GW, Romanelli AJ, Rossbacher JC, Moore IK, Regittnig W, Munoz DS, Kim JH, and Shulman GI. "n-3 Fatty acids preserve insulin sensitivity in vivo in a peroxisome proliferator-activated receptor-alpha-dependent manner." *Diabetes* 56 (2007): 1034–1041.

Neschen S, Morino K, Rossbacher JC, Pongratz RL, Cline GW, Sono S, Gillum M, and Shulman GI. "Fish oil regulates adiponectin secretion by a peroxisome proliferator-activated receptor-gamma-dependent mechanism in mice." *Diabetes* 55 (2006): 924–928.

Nieves D and Moreno JJ. "Role of 5-lipoxygenase pathway in the regulation of RAW 264.7 macrophage proliferation." *Biochemical Pharmacology* 72 (2006): 1022–1030.

Peres CM, Aronoff DM, Serezani CH, Flamand N, Faccioli LH, and Peters-Golden M. "Specific leukotriene receptors couple to distinct G proteins to effect stimulation of alveolar macrophage host defense functions." *The Journal of Immunology* 179 (2007): 5454–5461.

Perez-Matute P, Perez-Echarri N, Martinez JA, Marti A, and Moreno-Aliaga MJ. "Eicosapentaenoic acid actions on adiposity and insulin resistance in control and high-fat-fed rats: role of apoptosis, adiponectin and tumour necrosis factor-alpha." *British Journal of Nutrition* 97 (2007): 389–398.

Permana PA, Menge C, and Reaven PD. "Macrophage-secreted factors induce adipocyte inflammation and insulin resistance." *Biochemical and Biophysical Research Communications* 341 (2006): 507–514.

Petersen KF, Befroy D, Dufour S, Dziura J, Ariyan C, Rothman DL, Di Pietro L, Cline GW, and Shulman GI. "Mitochondrial dysfunction in the elderly: possible role in insulin resistance." *Science* 300 (2003): 1140–1142.

Pincelli AI, Brunani A, Scacchi M, Dubini A, Borsotti R, Tibaldi A, Pasqualinotto L, Maestri E, and Cavagnini F. "The serum concentration of tumor necrosis factor alpha is not an index of growth-hormone- or obesity-induced insulin resistance." *Hormone Research* 55 (2001): 57–64.

Pittas AG, Joseph NA, and Greenberg AS. "Adipocytokines and insulin resistance." *Journal of Clinical Endocrinology and Metabolism* 89 (2004): 447–452.

Bibliography

Poitout V and Robertson RP. "Glucolipotoxicity: Fuel excess and beta-cell dysfunction." *Endocrine Reviews* 29 (2008): 351–366.

Ramakers JD, Mensink RP, Schaart G, and Plat J. "Arachidonic acid but not eicosapentaenoic acid (EPA) and oleic acid activates NF-kappaB and elevates ICAM-1 expression in Caco-2 cells." *Lipids* 42 (2007): 687–698.

Rasouli N, Molavi B, Elbein SC, and Kern PA. "Ectopic fat accumulation and metabolic syndrome." *Diabetes, Obesity and Metabolism* 9 (2007): 1–10.

Reaven GM. "All obese individuals are not created equal: Insulin resistance is the major determinant of cardiovascular disease in overweight/obese individuals." *Diabetes and Vascular Disease Research* 2 (2005): 105–112.

Reaven GM and Laws A. *Insulin Resistance: The Metabolic Syndrome X.* Totowa, NJ: Humana Press, 1999.

Ruan H and Lodish HF. "Insulin resistance in adipose tissue: direct and indirect effects of tumor necrosis factor-alpha." *Cytokine and Growth Factor Reviews* 14 (2003): 447–455.

Sbarbati A, Osculati F, Silvagni D, Benati D, Galie M, Camoglio FS, Rigotti G, and Maffeis C. "Obesity and inflammation: evidence for an elementary lesion." *Pediatrics* 117 (2006): 220–223.

Sears B. *The Anti-Aging Zone.* New York: Regan Books, 1999.

Serhan CN. "Resolution phase of inflammation: novel endogenous anti-inflammatory and proresolving lipid mediators and pathways." *Annual Review of Immunology* 25 (2007): 101–137.

Serhan CN, Arita M, Hong S, and Gotlinger K. "Resolvins, docosatrienes, and neuroprotectins, novel omega-3-derived mediators, and their endogenous aspirin-triggered epimers." *Lipids* 39 (2004): 1125–1132.

Shi H, Kokoeva MV, Inouye K, Tzameli I, Yin H, Flier JS. "TLR4 links innate immunity and fatty acid-induced insulin resistance." *Journal of Clinical Investigation* 116 (2006): 3015–3025.

Shoelson SE, Lee J, and Goldfine AB. "Inflammation and insulin resistance." *Journal of Clinical Investigation* 116 (2006): 1793–1801.

Shoelson SE, Lee J, and Yuan M. "Inflammation and the IKK beta/I kappa B/NF-kappaB axis in obesity- and diet-induced insulin resistance." *International Journal of Obesity and Related Metabolic Disorders* 3 (2003): S49–52.

Song M, Kim K, Yoon JM, and Kim JB. "Activation of Toll-like receptor 4 is associated with insulin resistance in adipocytes." *Biochemical and Biophysical Research Communications* 346 (2006): 739–745.

Storlien LH, Kraegen EW, Chisholm DJ, Ford GL, Bruce DG, and Pascoe WS. "Fish oil prevents insulin resistance induced by high-fat feeding in rats." *Science* 237 (1987): 885–888.

Strissel KJ, Stancheva Z, Miyoshi H, Perfield JW, De Furia J, Jick Z, Greenberg AS, and Obin MS. "Adipocyte death, adipose tissue remodeling, and obesity complications." *Diabetes* 56 (2007): 2910–2918.

Todoric J, Loffler M, Huber J, Bilban M, Reimers M, Kadl A, Zeyda M, Waldhausl W, and Stulnig TM. "Adipose tissue inflammation induced by high-fat diet in obese diabetic mice is prevented by n-3 polyunsaturated fatty acids." *Diabetologia* 49 (2006): 2109–2119.

Trowbridge HO and Emling RC. *Inflammation: A Review of the Process—5th Edition*. Chicago: Quintessence Books, 1997.

Unger RH. "Lipotoxic diseases." *Annual Review of Medicine* 53 (2002): 319–336.

Weisberg SP, McCann D, Desai M, Rosenbaum M, Leibel RL, and Ferrante AW. "Obesity is associated with macrophage accumulation in adipose tissue." *Journal of Clinical Investigation* 112 (2003): 1796–1808.

Wellen KE and Hotamisligil GS. "Obesity-induced inflammatory changes in adipose tissue." *Journal of Clinical Investigation* 112 (2003): 1785–1788.

Xu H, Barnes GT, Yang Q, Tan G, Yang D, Chou CJ, Sole J, Nichols A, Ross JS, Tartaglia LA, and Chen H. "Chronic inflammation in fat plays a crucial role in the development of obesity-related insulin resistance." *Journal of Clinical Investigation* 112 (2003): 1821–1830.

Ye Y, Nishi SP, Manickavasagam S, Lin Y, Huang MH, Perez-Polo JR, Uretsky BF, and Birnbaum Y. "Activation of peroxisome proliferator-activated receptor-gamma (PPAR-gamma) by atorvastatin is mediated by 15-deoxy-delta-12,14-PGJ2." *Prostaglandins and Other Lipid Mediators* 84 (2007): 43–53.

Yeaman SJ. "Hormone-sensitive lipase—new roles for an old enzyme." *Biochemical Journal* 379 (2004): 11–22.

Bibliography

Appendix G—Nutrigenomics: How Diet Affects the Expression of Your Genes

Baur JA, Pearson KJ, Price NL, Jamieson HA, Lerin C, Kalra A, Prabhu VV, Allard JS, Lopez-Lluch G, Lewis K, Pistell PJ, Poosala S, Becker KG, Boss O, Gwinn D, Wang M, Ramaswamy S, Fishbein KW, Spencer RG, Lakatta EG, Le Couteur D, Shaw RJ, Navas P, Puigserver P, Ingram DK, de Cabo R, and Sinclair DA. "Resveratrol improves health and survival of mice on a high-calorie diet." *Nature* 444 (2006): 337–342.

Biesalski HK. "Polyphenols and inflammation: basic interactions." *Current Opinion in Clinical Nutrition and Metabolic Care* 10 (2007): 724–728.

Cai D, Yuan M, Frantz DF, Melendez PA, Hansen L, Lee J, and Shoelson SE. "Local and systemic insulin resistance resulting from hepatic activation of IKK-beta and NF-kappaB." *Nature Medicine* 11 (2005): 183–190.

Carluccio MA, Siculella L, Ancora MA, Massaro M, Scoditti E, Storelli C, Visioli F, Distante A, and De Caterina R. "Olive oil and red wine antioxidant polyphenols inhibit endothelial activation: antiatherogenic properties of Mediterranean diet phytochemicals." *Arteriosclerosis, Thrombosis, and Vascular Biology* 23 (2003): 622–629.

Chang JW, Kim CS, Kim SB, Park SK, Park JS, and Lee SK. "C-reactive protein induces NF-kappaB activation through intracellular calcium and ROS in human mesangial cells." *Nephron Experimental Nephrology* 101 (2005): e165–172.

Chiang N, Bermudez EA, Ridker PM, Hurwitz S, and Serhan CN. "Aspirin triggers anti-inflammatory 15-epi-lipoxin A4 and inhibits thromboxane in a randomized human trial." *Proceedings of the National Academy of Sciences (USA)* 101 (2004): 15178–15183.

Chiang N, Hurwitz S, Ridker PM, and Serhan CN. "Aspirin has a gender-dependent impact on anti-inflammatory 15-epi-lipoxin A4 formation: a randomized human trial." *Arteriosclerosis, Thrombosis, and Vascular Biology* 26 (2006): e14–17.

Collins T and Cybulsky ML. "NF-kappaB: pivotal mediator or innocent bystander in atherogenesis?" *Journal of Clinical Investigation* 107 (2001): 255–264.

Denys A, Hichami A, and Khan NA. "N-3 PUFAs modulate T-cell activation via protein kinase C-alpha and -epsilon and the NF-kappaB signaling pathway." *Journal of Lipid Research* 46 (2005): 752–758.

Esmaillzadeh A, Kimiagar M, Mehrabi Y, Azadbakht L, Hu FB, and Willett WC. "Fruit and vegetable intakes, C-reactive protein, and the metabolic syndrome." *American Journal of Clinical Nutrition* 84 (2006): 1489–1497.

Hughes-Fulford M, Li CF, Boonyaratanakornkit J, and Sayyah S. "Arachidonic acid activates phosphatidylinositol 3-kinase signaling and induces gene expression in prostate cancer." *Cancer Research* 66 (2006): 1427–1433.

Kim SR, Lee KS, Park HS, Park SJ, Min KH, Jin SM, and Lee YC. "Involvement of IL-10 in peroxisome proliferator-activated receptor gamma-mediated anti-inflammatory response in asthma." *Molecular Pharmacology* 68 (2005): 1568–1575.

Lagouge M, Argmann C, Gerhart-Hines Z, Meziane H, Lerin C, Daussin F, Messadeq N, Milne J, Lambert P, Elliott P, Geny B, Laakso M, Puigserver P, and Auwerx J. "Resveratrol improves mitochondrial function and protects against metabolic disease by activating SIRT1 and PGC-1alpha." *Cell* 127 (2006): 1109–1122.

Lawrence JR, Peter R, Baxter GJ, Robson J, Graham AB, and Paterson JR. "Urinary excretion of salicylate and salicylic acids by non-vegetarians, vegetarians, and patients taking low dose aspirin." *Journal of Clinical Pathology* 56 (2003): 651–653.

Lee JY, Plakidas A, Lee WH, Heikkinen A, Chanmugam P, Bray G, Hwang DH. "Differential modulation of Toll-like receptors by fatty acids: Preferential inhibition by n-3 polyunsaturated fatty acids." *Journal of Lipid Research* 44 (2003): 479–486.

Lee JY, Ye J, Gao Z, Youn HS, Lee WH, Zhao L, Sizemore N, and Hwang DH. "Reciprocal modulation of Toll-like receptor-4 signaling pathways involving MyD88 and phosphatidylinositol 3-kinase/AKT by saturated and polyunsaturated fatty acids." *Journal of Biological Chemistry* 278 (2003): 37041–37051.

Lee JY, Zhao L, Youn HS, Weatherill AR, Tapping R, Feng L, Lee WH, Fitzgerald KA, and Hwang DH. "Saturated fatty acid activates but polyunsaturated fatty acid inhibits Toll-like receptor 2 dimerized with Toll-like receptor 6 or 1." *Journal of Biological Chemistry* 279 (2004): 16971–1679.

Li H, Ruan XZ, Powis SH, Fernando R, Mon WY, Wheeler DC, Moorhead JF, and Varghese Z. "EPA and DHA reduce LPS-induced inflammation responses in HK-2 cells: evidence for a PPAR-gamma-dependent mechanism." *Kidney International* 67 (2005): 867–874.

McCarty MF. "Potential utility of natural polyphenols for reversing fat-induced insulin resistance." *Medical Hypotheses* 64 (2005): 628–635.

Nam NH. "Naturally occurring NF-kappaB inhibitors." *Mini Reviews in Medicinal Chemistry* 6 (2006): 945–951.

Novak TE, Babcock TA, Jho DH, Helton WS, and Espat NJ. "NF-kappaB inhibition by omega-3 fatty acids modulates LPS-stimulated macrophage TNF-alpha transcription."

Bibliography

American Journal Physiology—Lung Cellular Molecular Physiology 284 (2003): L84–89.

Paterson TJ, Baxter G, Lawrence J, Duthie G. "Is there a role for dietary salicylates in health?" *Proceedings of the Nutrition Society* 65 (2006): 93–96.

Ross JA, Maingay JP, Fearon KC, Sangster K, and Powell JJ. "Eicosapentaenoic acid perturbs signaling via the NF-kappaB transcriptional pathway in pancreatic tumour cells." *International Journal of Oncology* 23(6) (2003): 1733–1738.

Schroeder F, Petrescu AD, Huang H, Atshaves BP, McIntosh AL, Martin GG, Hosteler HA, Vespa A, Landrock D, Landrock KK, Payne HR, and Kier AB. "Role of fatty acid binding protein and long chain fatty acids in modulating nuclear receptors and gene transcription." *Lipids* 43 (2008): 1–17.

Serhan CN, Arita M, Hong S, and Gotlinger K. "Resolvins, docosatrienes, and neuro-protectins, novel omega-3-derived mediators, and their endogenous aspirin-triggered epimers." *Lipids* 39 (2004): 1125–1132.

Shoelson SE, Lee J, and Yuan M. "Inflammation and the IKK beta/I kappa B/NF-kappaB axis in obesity- and diet-induced insulin resistance." *International Journal of Obesity and Related Metabolic Disorders* 27 (2003): S49–52.

Suchankova G, Tekle M, Saha AK, Ruderman NB, Clarke SD, and Getty TW. "Dietary polyunsaturated fatty acids enhance hepatic AMP-activated protein kinase activity in rats." *Biochemical and Biophysical Research Communications* 326 (2005): 851–858.

Suganami T, Tanimoto-Koyama K, Nishida J, Itoh M, Yuan X, Mizuarai S, Kotani H, Yamaoka S, Miyake K, Aoe S, Kamei Y, and Ogawa Y. "Role of the Toll-like receptor 4/NF-kappaB pathway in saturated fatty acid-induced inflammatory changes in the interaction between adipocytes and macrophages." *Arteriosclerosis, Thrombosis, and Vascular Biology* 27 (2007): 84–91.

Yoon JH and Baek SJ. "Molecular targets of dietary polyphenols with anti-inflammatory properties." *Yonsei Medical Journal* 46 (2005): 585–596.

Youn HS, Lee JY, Saitoh SI, Miyake K, Kang KW, Choi YJ, and Hwang DH. "Suppression of MyD88 and TRIF-dependent signaling pathways of Toll-like receptor by epigallocatechin-3-gallate, a polyphenol component of green tea." *Biochemical Pharmacology* 72 (2006): 850–859.

Youn HS, Saitoh SI, Miyake K, and Hwang DH. "Inhibition of homodimerization of Toll-like receptor 4 by curcumin." *Biochemical Pharmacology* 72(1) (2006): 62–69.

Zang M, Xu S, Maitland-Toolan KA, Zuccollo A, Hou X, Jiang B, Wierzbicki M, Verbeuren TJ, and Cohen RA. "Polyphenols stimulate AMP-activated protein kinase, lower lipids, and inhibit accelerated atherosclerosis in diabetic LDL receptor-deficient mice." *Diabetes* 55 (2006): 2180–2191.

Zhao Y, Joshi-Barve S, Barve S, and Chen LH. "Eicosapentaenoic acid prevents LPS-induced TNF-alpha expression by preventing NF-kappaB activation." *Journal of the American College of Nutrition* 23 (2004): 71–78.

Appendix H—Zone Food Blocks

Sears B. *A Week in the Zone.* New York: Regan Books, 2000.

———. *Mastering the Zone.* New York: Regan Books, 1997.

———. *The Anti-Inflammation Zone.* New York: Regan Books, 2005.

———. *The Zone.* New York: Regan Books, 1995.

———. *What to Eat in the Zone.* New York: Regan Books, 2003.

———. *Zone Food Blocks.* New York: Regan Books, 1998.

———. *Zone Perfect Meals in Minutes.* New York: Regan Books, 1997.

Sears B and Sears L. *Zone Meals in Seconds.* New York: Regan Books, 2004.

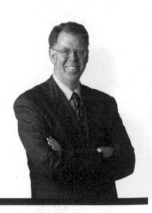

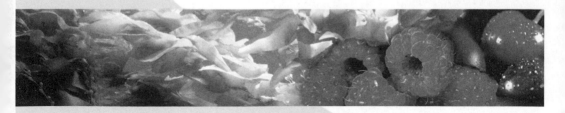